Lean and Green Cookbook for Beginners 2022

Over 1200 Days of Fueling Hacks and Lean and Green Recipes That Burn Body Fat and Get You to Lose Weight.
Two Different Meal Plans Included: 5&1 and 4&2&1.

Isabel Taylor

© **Copyright 2022 - All rights reserved.**

This document is geared towards providing exact and reliable information in regard to the topic and issue covered.

- From a Declaration of Principles which was accepted and approved equally by a Committee of the American Bar Association and a Committee of Publishers and Associations.

In no way is it legal to reproduce, duplicate, or transmit any part of this document in either electronic means or in printed format. All rights reserved.

The information provided herein is stated to be truthful and consistent, in that any liability, in terms of inattention or otherwise, by any usage or abuse of any policies, processes, or directions contained within is the solitary and utter responsibility of the recipient reader. Under no circumstances will any legal responsibility or blame be held against the publisher for any reparation, damages, or monetary loss due to the information herein, either directly or indirectly.

Respective authors own all copyrights not held by the publisher.

The information herein is offered for informational purposes solely and is universal as so. The presentation of the information is without contract or any type of guarantee assurance.

The trademarks that are used are without any consent, and the publication of the trademark is without permission or backing by the trademark owner. All trademarks and brands within this book are for clarifying purposes only and are owned by the owners themselves, not affiliated with this document.

TABLE OF CONTENTS

INTRODUCTION 11

WHAT THE LEAN AND GREEN DIET IS? 12
- 154. Who should try it? 12
- 155. Foods to Eat on a Lean and Green Diet 13
- 156. What is Fueling? 14
- 157. Foods to Avoid 14
- 158. How Does Lean and Green Diet Work for Weight Loss? 15

FUELING HACKS RECIPES 16
- 159. Parmesan Zucchini Rounds 16
- 160. Green Bean Casserole 16
- 161. Zucchini Spaghetti 16
- 162. Cabbage and Radishes Mix 17
- 163. Kale Chips 17
- 164. Coriander Artichokes 17
- 165. Spinach and Artichokes Sauté 18
- 166. Green Beans 18
- 167. Balsamic Cabbage 18
- 168. Herbed Radish Sauté 18
- 169. Roasted Tomatoes 19
- 170. Kale and Walnuts 19
- 171. Bok Choy and Butter Sauce 19
- 172. Turmeric Mushroom 20
- 173. Berry Mojito 20
- 174. Coconut Smoothie 20
- 175. Tiramisu Shake 21
- 176. Vanilla Shake 21
- 177. Shamrock Shake 21
- 178. Chocolate Shake 21
- 179. Peppermint Mocha 22
- 180. Pumpkin Frappe 22
- 181. Vanilla Frappe 22
- 182. Chocolate Frappe 23
- 183. Caramel Macchiato Frappe 23
- 184. Eggnog 23
- 185. Pumpkin Spiced Latte 24
- 186. Hot Chocolate 24
- 187. Cherry Mocha Popsicles 24
- 188. Yogurt Cookie Dough 25
- 189. Chocolate Coconut Pie 25
- 190. Caramel Crunch Parfait 25
- 191. Chocolate Berry Parfait 26
- 192. Brownie Pudding 26
- 193. Brownie Peanut Butter Pudding 26
- 194. Chia Seed Pudding 27
- 195. Chocolate Cake Fries 27
- 196. French Toast Sticks 27

#	Title	Page
197.	Fudge Balls	28
198.	Peanut Butter Bites	28
199.	Yogurt Cereal Bark	28
200.	Chocolate Crunch Cookies	29
201.	Oatmeal Cookies	29
202.	Peanut Butter Cookies	29
203.	Mint Cookies	30
204.	Gingersnap Cookies	30
205.	Crunch Sandwich Cookies	31
206.	Sandwich Cookies	31
207.	Snickerdoodles	32
208.	Chocolate Whoopie Pies	32
209.	Brownie Bites	33
210.	Chocolate Haystacks	33

BREAKFAST RECIPES 34

#	Title	Page
211.	Gluten-Free Pancakes	34
212.	Mushroom & Spinach Omelet	34
213.	Pizza Hack	34
214.	Sweet Cashew Cheese Spread	35
215.	Mini Zucchini Bites	35
216.	Whole-Wheat Blueberry Muffins	36
217.	Hemp Seed Porridge	36
218.	Walnut Crunch Banana Bread	36
219.	Plant-Powered Pancakes	37
220.	Mini Mac in a Bowl	37
221.	Shake Cake Fueling	38
222.	Biscuit Pizza	38
223.	Lean and Green Smoothie 1	38
224.	Lean and Green Smoothie 2	39
225.	Lean and Green Chicken Pesto Pasta	39
226.	Open-Face Egg Sandwiches with Cilantro-Jalapeño Spread	39
227.	Alkaline Blueberry Spelt Pancakes	40
228.	Alkaline Blueberry Muffins	40
229.	Crunchy Quinoa Meal	41
230.	Coconut Pancakes	41
231.	Cashew Yogurt Bowl	42
232.	Zucchini Breakfast Bars	42
233.	Cheesy Scrambled Tofu	42
234.	Zucchini Bacon Bake	43
235.	Cauliflower Breakfast Casserole	43
236.	Jalapeno Breakfast Casserole	44
237.	Easy Cheese Egg Bake	44
238.	Sausage Egg Omelet	44
239.	Broccoli Egg Bake	45
240.	Chicken Cheese Quiche	45
241.	Egg & Bacon Cups	45
242.	Cottage Cheese Hotcake	46
243.	Chard Omelet	46
244.	Scrambled Pesto Eggs	47
245.	Devil Eggs	47
246.	Asparagus & Crabmeat Frittata	47
247.	Bacon Cheeseburger	48
248.	Ancho Tilapia on Cauliflower Rice	48
249.	Turkey Caprese Meatloaf Cups	49

250. Cinnamon Coconut Porridge 49

LUNCH RECIPES 50

251. Bacon-Wrapped Asparagus.................50
252. Spinach Chicken 50
253. Lemongrass Prawns.....................50
254. Stuffed Mushrooms 51
255. Keto Zucchini Pizza 51
256. Crab Cakes 52
257. Low Carb Black Beans Chili Chicken .52
258. Quick Keto BLT Chicken Salad 52
259. Quick Healthy Avocado Tuna Salad...53
260. Flavorful Keto Taco Soup.................53
261. Delicious Instant Pot Keto Buffalo Chicken Soup 54
262. Creamy Low Carb Cream of Mushroom Soup 54
263. Easy Keto Chicken Soup 54
264. Taco Casserole 55
265. Quick Keto Roasted Tomato Soup.....55
266. Delicious Low Carb Chicken Caesar Salad 56
267. Keto Cheesy Broccoli Soup 56
268. Creamy Low Carb Zucchini Alfredo ...56
269. Amazing Low Carb Shrimp Lettuce Wraps. 57
270. Tasty Low Carb Cucumber Salad 57
271. Classic Low Carb Cobb Salad 58
272. Yummy Keto Mushroom Asparagus Frittata...58
273. Yogurt Garlic Chicken........................59

274. Grilled Ham & Cheese 59
275. Prosciutto Spinach Salad 60
276. Riced Cauliflower & Curry Chicken ...60
277. Mashed Garlic Turnips 60
278. Lasagna Spaghetti Squash................61
279. Blue Cheese Chicken Wedges 61
280. 'Oh so good' Salad............................61
281. 'I Love Bacon' 62
282. Lemon Dill Trout................................62
283. Meatballs Curry................................62
284. Pork with Veggies 63
285. Pork Taco Bake 64
286. Spinach Pie 64
287. Baked Chicken Fajitas 65
288. Pesto Zucchini Noodles 65
289. Sautéed Crispy Zucchini 65

DINNER RECIPES 66

290. Zucchini Salmon Salad......................66
291. Pan Fried Salmon..............................66
292. Grilled Salmon with Pineapple Salsa .66
293. Mediterranean Chickpea Salad..........67
294. Warm Chorizo Chickpea Salad 67
295. Jalapeno Lentil Burgers 67
296. Grandma's Rice................................68
297. Baked Beef Zucchini 69
298. Baked Tuna with Asparagus 69
299. Lamb Stuffed Avocado 70

300.	Mozzarella Sticks	70
301.	Greek Roasted Fish	71
302.	Tomato Fish Bake	71
303.	Garlicky Tomato Chicken Casserole	71
304.	Chicken Cacciatore	72
305.	Fennel Wild Rice Risotto	72
306.	Wild Rice Prawn Salad	72
307.	Chicken Broccoli Salad with Avocado Dressing	73
308.	Seafood Paella	73
151.	Herbed Roasted Chicken Breasts	74
152.	Marinated Chicken Breasts	74
153.	Greek Style Quesadillas	74
309.	Creamy Penne	75
310.	Light Paprika Moussaka	75
311.	Cucumber Container with Spices and Greek Yogurt	76
312.	Stuffed Bell Peppers with Quinoa	76
313.	Mediterranean Burrito	76
314.	Sweet Potato Bacon Mash	77
315.	Prosciutto Wrapped Mozzarella Balls	77
316.	Garlic Chicken Balls	77
317.	Monkey Salad	78
318.	Jarlsberg Lunch Omelet	78
319.	Fiery Jalapeno Poppers	78
320.	Bacon & Chicken Patties	79
321.	Cheddar Bacon Burst	79
322.	Quinoa with Vegetables	80
323.	Chicken Goulash	80
324.	Chicken & Turkey Meatloaf	80

DESSERT RECIPES ... 82

325.	Mint chocolate pudding cookies	82
326.	Tasty Pecan Pie Muffins	82
327.	Yummy Lime Pie	83
328.	Fresh Green Grape Salad	83
329.	Broccoli Cheese Waffles	83
330.	Hearty Fruit Salad	84
331.	Vegan Waffles with Kale	84
332.	Best Chia Pudding	85
333.	Sweet Potato Muffins	85
334.	Gingerbread Biscotti	86
335.	Sweet Pumpkin Waffles	86
336.	Chia Pudding	87
337.	Avocado Pudding	87
338.	Smooth Peanut Butter Cream	87
339.	Raspberry Ice Cream	88
340.	Chocolate Frosty	88
341.	Bounty Bars	88
342.	Delicious Brownie Bites	89
343.	Chocolate Popsicle	89
344.	Pumpkin Balls	89
345.	Blueberry Muffins	90
346.	Vanilla Avocado Popsicles	90
347.	Chocolate Almond Butter Brownie	90
348.	Peanut Butter Fudge	91
349.	Almond Butter Fudge	91

350. Optavia Granola 91
351. Peanut Butter Brownie 92
352. Chocolate Cherry Cookie 92
353. Stuffed pears with almonds 92
354. Peanut Butter Cups 93
355. Medifast Rolls 93
356. Apple Crisp 93
357. Cherry Dessert 94
358. Vanilla Pudding 94

SNACK RECIPES 96

359. Sausage and Cheese Dip 96
360. Stuffed Avocado 96
361. Tasty Onion and Cauliflower Dip 96
362. Avocado Taco Boat 97
363. Pesto Crackers 97
364. Chicken and Mushrooms 98
365. Marinated Eggs 98
366. Chili Mango and Watermelon Salsa ... 98
367. Pumpkin Muffins 99
368. Chicken Enchilada Bake 99
369. Greek Tuna Salad Bites 100
370. Veggie Fritters 100
371. Cucumber Sandwich Bites 100
372. White Bean Dip 101
373. Eggplant Dip 101
374. Feta Artichoke Dip 101
375. Avocado Dip 102
376. Green Beans Rice 102
377. Garlic Kale 102
378. Celery and Green Beans Mix 102
379. Parmesan Asparagus 103
380. Ginger Kale 103
381. Spicy Red Cabbage 103

APPETIZER RECIPES 104

382. Salmon Burger 104
383. Salmon Sandwich with Avocado and Egg 104
384. Spinach and Cottage Cheese Sandwich 104
385. Feta and Pesto Wrap 105
386. Cheese and Onion on Bagel 105
387. Bananas in Nut Cups 105
388. Apple Salad Sandwich 106
389. Buttermilk Ice Cream Shake 106
390. Buttermilk Shake 106
391. Cantaloupe Orange Milk Shakes 107
392. Cheese on Rye Bread 107
393. Buckwheat Granola 107
394. Apple Pancakes 108
395. Matcha Pancakes 108
396. Smoked Salmon & Kale Scramble 108
397. Kale & Mushroom Frittata 109
398. Kale, Apple, & Cranberry Salad 109
399. Arugula, Strawberry, & Orange Salad 109
400. Lean and Green Crockpot Chili 110

SOUPS AND SALADS RECIPES 111

- 401. California Soup 111
- 402. Cheesy Cauliflower Soup 111
- 403. Egg drop Soup 111
- 404. Cauliflower, Spinach, and Cheese Soup 112
- 405. Corner-Filling Soup 112
- 406. Stracciatella 112
- 407. Peanut Soup 113
- 408. Soap De Frijoles Negros 113
- 409. Artichoke Soup 114
- 410. Curried Pumpkin Soup 114
- 411. Cheesy Onion Soup 115
- 412. Cream of Potato Soup 115
- 413. Swiss cheese and Broccoli Soup 116
- 414. Tavern Soup 116
- 415. Broccoli Blue Cheese Soup 116
- 416. Cream of Mushroom Soup 117
- 417. Olive Soup 117
- 418. Wasabi Tuna Asian Salad 118
- 419. Lemon Greek Salad 118
- 420. Broccoli Salad 118
- 421. Potato Carrot Salad 119
- 422. Marinated Veggie Salad 119
- 423. Mediterranean Salad 120
- 424. Potato Tuna Salad 120
- 425. High Protein Salad 120
- 426. Pea Salad 121
- 427. Snap Pea Salad 121
- 428. Cucumber Tomato Chopped Salad .. 121
- 429. Zucchini Pasta Salad 122
- 430. Egg Avocado Salad 122
- 431. Asian Cabbage Salad 122
- 432. Tangy Kale Salad 123
- 433. Crunchy Cauliflower Salad 123
- 434. Crisp Summer Cucumber Salad 124

AIR FRYER RECIPES 125

- 435. Air Fryer Italian Pork Chops 125
- 436. Air Fried Riblets 125
- 437. Pork Tenderloin with Fried Bell Peppers 125
- 438. Air Fried Beef Jerky 125
- 439. Air Fried Pot Roast 126
- 440. Mexican-Style Air Fryer Stuffed Chicken Breasts 126
- 441. Mixed Vegetables with Chicken 126
- 442. Low Carb Parmesan Chicken Meatballs 127
- 443. Sriracha-honey Chicken Wings 127
- 444. Orange Chicken Wings 128
- 445. Air Fryer Catfish with Cajun Seasoning 128
- 446. Air Fryer Sushi Roll 128
- 447. Air Fryer Garlic-Lime Shrimp Kebabs 129
- 448. Fish Finger Sandwich 129
- 449. Healthy Air Fryer Tuna Patties 129
- 450. Cheese Broccoli Fritters 130

451. Air Fryer Bell Peppers 130	Week 4 136
452. Air Fried Tasty Eggplant 130	**MEAL PLAN 4&2&1 ...... 137**
453. Asian Green Beans 131	Week 1 137
454. Spicy Asian Brussels Sprouts 131	Week 2 138
455. Taco Salad 131	Week 3 139
456. Yogurt Trail Mix Bars 131	Week 4 140
457. Curried Tuna Salad 132	**CONCLUSION 141**
MEAL PLAN 5&1 133	**MEASUREMENT CONVERSION 142**
Week 1 133	**INDEX 143**
Week 2 134	
Week 3 135	

INTRODUCTION

In recent days, more and more people are becoming aware of the term "Lean and Green Diet." This diet is a mixture of veganism, a majoritarian desire to live in harmony with nature, and an emphasis on "clean eating" in the form of raw foods. The results: increased energy levels, better skin and hair quality, decreased weight gain, etc.

The Lean and Green Diet is a healthy yet appetizing meal that will help you lose weight as well as keep you energized throughout the day. To start with this diet, try out pantry staples such as rosemary sprigs or thyme sprigs for flavor. If you are a meat-eater, then you can always add some kind of protein—turkey, chicken, or tofu.

Another key part of lean and green meals is the salads. Start your day with a salad for example a salad with spinach, cucumber, and tomato. Also try out various kinds of apple cores: sliced apples with some olive oil on them or grated apples. You need to eat lots of fruits and vegetables to maintain your weight—fruits and vegetables are low in calories yet they pack in many vitamins and they are also loaded with fiber which will make you feel full faster thereby controlling your appetite.

You should drink more water as it is essential for proper function as well as proper digestion. You need to drink at least 64 fluid oz. of water a day. By drinking lots of water, you will be able to shed your fat even more effectively by flushing excess water out of your body.

You should also include some spices in your diet such as ginger, turmeric, and cinnamon for taste. You can also add certain herbs to increase your metabolism or detoxify your body. For example, if you are cleansing or not feeling well, then you can add some nettle or dandelion or burdock root for an energy boost and a detoxification purpose.

The Lean and Green Diet is part of a healthy lifestyle and you must include certain tools for your success. You should always have some kind of journal or book to keep track of your progress as well as keep you motivated. A healthy environment is also important as a living environment. In fact, the environment is one of the strongest factors of weight management. The right lighting will make you feel better while being in a dark room makes you feel sluggish and unhealthy—especially if it's too cold outside.

It is best to keep your refrigerator organized to eliminate over-eating. You should also purchase smaller plates to control your intake of food. You should always maintain a water bottle and glass of water with yourself as well so that you don't rely on other drinks that are high in calories or sugar.

The Lean and Green Diet is a diet with no restrictions or limitations and it helps you reach your weight loss goals while making sure that you stay healthy throughout the process. This diet includes many varieties of foods that are tasty and healthy at the same time. The key to staying fit is proper nutrition, exercise, motivation, and keeping track of your progress.

WHAT THE LEAN AND GREEN DIET IS?

The lean and green diet is one of the most nutritious diets out there. It's meant to be more environmentally friendly than other diets like veganism and vegetarianism, but still, provides good nutrition for your body. The main principle behind this diet is to focus on whole foods that have minimal processing, are raw or cooked at low temperatures, and avoid foods with a lot of chemicals.

This diet makes you feel good both physically and mentally as it promotes health in a nontoxic way.

154. Who should try it?

People who have the time and resources to support this diet should, because like with any diet, it requires a significant amount of time and personal power. If you have the chance to do some home cooking or would rather not shop in supermarkets that sell processed foods, this is an excellent way to live a healthy lifestyle. You could also try it merely as a change in some aspects of your everyday life, or as an addition to other diets if you are on a restricted budget.

Lean and Green is a diet program that involves a combination of fresh foods, and pre-prepared foods and snacks. Lean and Green also offers additional help from a designated support person. Once you have completed your twelve-week start-up plan, your average Lean and Green meal should then include five to seven ounces of cooked lean protein, plus three servings of non-starchy vegetables, and up to two servings of healthy fats. The plan is to eat up to six meals throughout the day.

If you wish to lose more weight than you lose in the first phase, you can stay on the initial diet plan longer, until you reach your target weight. Once you have reached that weight, you should safely enter the "transition phase." This involves slowly increasing your overall daily food intake to no more than 1,550 calories per day while adding a wider variety of foods, which will include whole grains, fruits, and low-fat dairy products such as yogurt and cheese. The Lean and Green diet also provides additional tools to aid weight loss and maintenance, which include tips and inspiration, community forums, weekly support calls, and an app that allows you to set meal reminders to track your food intake and your activity level.

In short, the Lean and Green diet is designed to help people lose weight and fat by reducing calories and carbs through portion-controlled meals and snacks. Its basis is to reduce carbs programs that combine processed, packaged calorie-counted foods with homemade meals which encourage weight loss. You can choose from several options, which all include products called "fuelings" as well as homemade meals, which follow the Lean and Green carb-fat ratio. The fuelings comprise over sixty items that are low in carbs, but high in protein and probiotic cultures. These friendly bacteria can boost your gut health. These fuelings include snack bars, cookies, shakes, puddings, cereals, soups, and pasta. All super-convenient and nutritious, while designed to help you feel satisfied.

155. <u>**Foods to Eat on a Lean and Green Diet**</u>

It's the first question that people always ask about a new diet: "What will I be eating?" Because food is important to us all. It is not only essential to our life, but it is also pleasurable and sociable. Most of us are used to eating a range of foods from all the essential groups, but we all have to confess that we have our favorites, and our pet hates! So, firstly, let me reassure you, by telling you what you won't be eating: there is nothing in the Lean and Green diet that is "weird," unusual, or just boring and unappetizing! You will be eating a huge selection of natural, nourishing foods; foods that you are already used to preparing and eating. The weight-loss secret lies in the planning, support, and execution of the program that you will be choosing to suit your needs and preferences.

The Lean and Green diet plan includes two weight loss programs, in addition to a carefully balanced weight maintenance plan. So, to answer this question: what you eat, how frequently you eat it, and how much of it you will be eating, depends totally on which of the plans you are on, and at which stage of the plan you are on at any given time.

A lot of diets that are on the market are successful only because they radically limit the types of food that you are allowed to eat, and how you can cook or combine them. Lean and Green doesn't do this, because we think that this way to eat can become rather boring eventually. So, now you don't have to worry about that, there are no unpleasant surprises in store when you choose to eat Lean and Green! The wide variety and the numerous styles of food that you will be enjoying will keep you feeling nourished and happy to continue. This specialized cookbook will help you to prepare and include all of the readily available, low-cost, popular foods which should always appear in any healthy diet. What's more, using Lean and Green, you will be eating a lot of familiar, nourishing, scrummy foods at selected intervals throughout the day, which will help you to enrich your body while you are losing excess unhealthy weight.

No limits on the amounts of greens and non-starchy vegetables that you consume either. You can tuck into cabbage, kale, cauliflower, broccoli, asparagus, and zucchini. You are not limited to fat-free food either. On this diet, you will be eating tasty foods which contain healthy fats. Fats like olive and nut oil for cooking and salad dressing are good. If you are not vegan, you will be able to eat lots of low-fat dairy foods. Yummy yogurts and tasty cheeses are not off-limits! Fresh eggs, low-fat milk, and frozen desserts are OK too. Lots of lovely fresh fruits are OK. Thumbs up to crisp apples, juicy oranges, sweet, grapes, zesty pineapples, and energizing bananas! Finally, to help to keep you feeling satisfied throughout the day, the Lean and Green diet naturally includes those comforting, life-giving, delicious essential whole grains and seeds. It's all well-balanced, convenient and it tastes good!

156. What is Fueling?

Fueling is a measured, calorie-controlled way of snacking, and it helps you to maintain your energy levels, as well as feel full throughout the day. More specifically, regular fuelings ensure that you are correctly nourished for your activity levels, whether you are working at your job, or working out. Correctly consumed fuelings provide you with the assurance that you won't be losing essential muscle mass while you are on the Lean and Green diet because, with carefully prepared fueling products, you'll be eating lots of the protein, fiber, and key nutrients that are essential to sustaining muscle mass.

157. Foods to Avoid

When you eat more healthily, there are foods that you need to cut out. It's the usual suspects: fats should be the healthy kind, so, butter, vegetable shortening, and coconut oil are not recommended. You should also limit the amounts of starchy vegetables you eat: corn, potatoes, peas, etc. Those with a sweet tooth: sugary drinks, desserts, cookies, and chocolate are all out.

As you know, it's not what you eat or when you eat that's crucial to weight loss. How often you eat is also an important aspect. Lean and green is no exception to this rule.

The eating habits and preferences that everyone has are as unique as their biology and personality. We are all creatures of habit. Some of our habits are good and some not so good! Some people enjoy eating at least one large meal every day, but they don't refuel in between times. They start their day with a hearty breakfast and eat frugally throughout the day. Some skip breakfast altogether, then have a quick snack for lunch, because they prefer to eat their main meal later. Some busy people are "grazers" who like to eat small, frequent meals. There is one group of people who snack all day long and never eat a balanced meal.

Eating habits and preferences for certain foods are totally a personal thing. There are carb-loaders, there are sugar cravers, some are into fatty foods, and some are more health-conscious, following plant-based diets. Some people have to adjust their habits when they go Lean and Green.

As I explained, the essence of the Lean and Green diet is to "fuel" your body regularly throughout the day, to supplement either one, two, or three main meals. The simplicity and versatility of the Lean and Green diet are really helpful. You can try out all three plans, to see which one best meets your needs, and continues to work well for you over time. Once you reach your target weight, you can experiment. The cookbook will help you to do this because it gives you recipes to prepare when you want to eat balanced, fresh food.

The Lean and Green diet advises that you eat six or seven times per day depending on the plan.

- **Optimal Weight 5 & 1 Plan.** This is the most popular plan, it includes five fuelings, and one balanced Lean and Green meal each day.

- **Optimal Weight 4 & 2 & 1 Plan.** This is for people who need more calories and flexibility in food choices. This includes four fuelings, two Lean and Green meals, and one snack per day.
- **Optimal Health 3 & 3 Plan.** It is specially designed for maintenance. It includes three fuelings and three balanced Lean and Green meals per day.

158. How Does Lean and Green Diet Work for Weight Loss?

The Lean and Green diet will work for you and support you if you want to lose excess weight and body fat and maintain the changes. One of the main reasons that the Lean and Green diet does work so efficiently is that the diet plan is so easy to implement and maintain, so you don't "fall off the wagon" and cheat yourself, by eating more than you should or foods that you shouldn't eat. The Lean and Green diet helps you to lose weight and cut your body fat because it is designed very precisely, to help you quickly get rid of those unwanted extra inches. It helps you to achieve this by reducing the calories and carbs that you eat every day, through the use of the carefully portion-controlled meals and snacks that are included in the program. If you are using these meals and snacks and combining them with a regular exercise regime, (and you are not cheating and snacking on chocolate!) the result that you achieve will be a substantial overall weight loss and improved health that you can easily maintain.

Over the last twenty years, weight loss has become an influential industry, with many diets and products on the market. So, necessarily, there has been a lot of clinical research into the efficiency and safety of weight loss products and diets. Some studies have clearly shown that greater weight loss is ensured if those who wish to lose weight follow a regime that contains either full or partial meal replacement plans, compared with more traditional calorie-restricted diets which do not contain any meal replacement products.

The bottom line is that by reducing your overall calorie intake, the Lean and Green diet is going to be very effective for weight loss. If you follow the Lean and Green diet, as per the recommendations, it makes changing your eating habits very easy to do. A comprehensive sixteen-week study of 198 people confirmed that the people who were on the Lean and Green 5 & 1 Plan had significantly lower weight, and body fat, as well as smaller waist circumferences, compared with the people who were in the control group, who were not on the Lean and Green diet. Most people on the 5 & 1 Plan lost 5.7% of their body weight, though 28.1% lost 10%.

Give the Lean and Green diet a try. Using this supporting cookbook, the only thing that you have to lose is weight!

FUELING HACKS RECIPES

159. Parmesan Zucchini Rounds

Difficulty: Easy
Preparation Time: 25 minutes
Cooking Time: 20 minutes
Servings: 4
Ingredients:
- 4 zucchinis; sliced
- 1 1/2 cups Parmesan; grated
- 1/4 cup parsley; chopped.
- 1 egg; whisked
- 1 egg white; whisked
- 1/2 tsp garlic powder
- Cooking spray

Directions:
1. Take a bowl and mix the egg with egg whites, Parmesan, parsley, and garlic powder. Then whisk.
2. Dredge each zucchini slice in this mix, place them all in your air fryer's basket, grease them with cooking spray and cook at 370°F for 20 minutes.
3. Divide between plates and serve as a side dish.

Nutrition:
- Calories: 183
- Fat: 6 g
- Fiber: 2 g
- Carbs: 3 g
- Protein: 8 g

160. Green Bean Casserole

Difficulty: Easy
Preparation Time: 25 minutes
Cooking Time: 20 minutes
Servings: 4
Ingredients:
- 1 lb. fresh green beans, edges trimmed
- 1/2 oz. pork rinds, finely ground
- 1 oz. full-fat cream cheese
- 1/2 cup heavy whipping cream.
- 1/4 cup yellow onion, diced
- 1/2 cup white mushrooms, chopped
- 1/2 cup chicken broth
- 1 tbsp unsalted butter
- 1/4 tsp xanthan gum

Directions:
1. Melt the butter in a preheated skillet.
2. Sauté the onion and mushrooms until soft and fragrant, for 3–5 minutes.
3. Add the heavy cream, cream cheese, and broth to the skillet. Lightly, beat until smooth. Boil and then simmer. Put the xanthan gum in the pan and remove it from heat.
4. Cut green beans into 2-inch pieces and place in a 4-cup round pan. Pour the sauce mixture over them and stir until covered. Fill the plate with ground pork rinds. Place in the fryer basket.
5. Set the temperature to 320°F and set the timer for 15 minutes. The top will be a golden and green bean fork when fully cooked. Serve hot.

Nutrition:
- Calories: 267
- Protein: 3.6 g
- Fat: 23.4 g
- Carbs: 9.7 g

161. Zucchini Spaghetti

Difficulty: Medium
Preparation Time: 20 minutes
Cooking Time: 15 minutes
Servings: 4
Ingredients:
- 1 lb. zucchinis, cut with a spiralizer
- 1 cup Parmesan, grated
- 1/4 cup parsley, chopped.
- 1/4 cup olive oil
- 2 garlic cloves; minced
- 1/2 tsp red pepper flakes
- Salt and black pepper to taste.

Directions:
1. In a pan that fits into your air fryer, mix all the ingredients, toss, put into the fryer and cook at 370°F for 15 minutes.
2. Divide between plates and serve as a side dish.

Nutrition:
- Calories: 200
- Fat: 6 g
- Carbs: 4 g
- Protein: 5 g

162. Cabbage and Radishes Mix

Difficulty: Easy
Preparation Time: 20 minutes
Cooking Time: 15 minutes
Servings: 4
Ingredients:
- 2 cups green cabbage; shredded
- 1/2 cup celery leaves; chopped.
- 1/4 cup green onions; chopped.
- 2 radishes; sliced
- 1 tbsp olive oil
- 1 tbsp balsamic vinegar
- 1/2 tsp hot paprika
- 1 tsp lemon juice

Directions:
1. In your air fryer's pan, combine all the ingredients and toss well.
2. Place the pan in the fryer and cook at 380°F for 15 minutes.
3. Divide between plates and serve as a side dish.

Nutrition:
- Calories: 130
- Fat: 4 g
- Carbs: 4 g
- Protein: 7 g

163. Kale Chips

Difficulty: Easy
Preparation Time: 10 minutes
Cooking Time: 5 minutes
Servings: 4
Ingredients:
- 2 cups stemmed kale
- 1/2 tsp salt
- 1 tsp avocado oil

Directions:
1. Take a large bowl, sprinkle the cabbage in avocado oil, and sprinkle with salt. Place in the fryer basket.
2. Set the temperature to 400°F and set the timer for 5 minutes. The kale will be crispy when done.
3. Serve immediately.

Nutrition:
- Calories: 25
- Protein: 0.5 g
- Fat: 2.2 g
- Carbs: 1.1 g

164. Coriander Artichokes

Difficulty: Intermediate
Preparation Time: 20 minutes
Cooking Time: 15 minutes
Servings: 4
Ingredients:
- 12 oz. artichoke hearts
- 1 tbsp lemon juice
- 1 tsp coriander, ground
- 1/2 tsp cumin seeds
- 1/2 tsp olive oil
- Salt and black pepper to taste

Directions:
1. In a pan that fits into your air fryer, mix all the ingredients, toss, put the pan into the fryer and cook at 370°F for 15 minutes.
2. Divide the mix between plates and serve as a side dish.

Nutrition:
- Calories: 200
- Fat: 7 g

- Carbs: 5 g
- Protein: 8 g

165. Spinach and Artichokes Sauté

Difficulty: Medium
Preparation Time: 20 minutes
Cooking Time: 15 minutes
Servings: 4
Ingredients:
- 10 oz. artichoke hearts; halved
- 3 cups baby spinach
- 3 garlic cloves
- 1/4 cup veggie stock
- 1 tsp lime juice
- Salt and black pepper to taste.

Directions:
1. In a pan that fits into your air fryer, mix all the ingredients, toss, put into the fryer and cook at 370°F for 15 minutes.
2. Divide between plates and serve as a side dish.

Nutrition:
- Calories: 209
- Fat: 6 g
- Carbs: 4 g
- Protein: 8 g

166. Green Beans

Difficulty: Easy
Preparation Time: 5 minutes
Cooking Time: 20 minutes
Servings: 4
Ingredients:
- 2 cups green beans; trimmed
- 1 tbsp hot paprika
- 1 tbsp olive oil
- A pinch of salt and black pepper

Directions:
1. Take a bowl and mix the green beans with the other ingredients, toss, put them in the air fryer's basket and cook at 370°F for 20 minutes.
2. Divide between plates and serve as a side dish.

Nutrition:
- Calories: 120
- Fat: 5 g
- Carbs: 4 g
- Protein: 2 g

167. Balsamic Cabbage

Difficulty: Easy
Preparation Time: 10 minutes
Cooking Time: 15 minutes
Servings: 4
Ingredients:
- 2 cups red cabbage, shredded
- 2 garlic cloves, minced
- 1 tbsp olive oil
- 1 tbsp balsamic vinegar
- Salt and black pepper to taste

Directions:
1. In a pan that fits into the air fryer, combine all the ingredients, toss, put the pan into the oven and cook at 380°F for 15 minutes.
2. Divide between plates and serve as a side dish.

Nutrition:
- Calories: 151
- Fat: 2 g
- Carbs: 5 g
- Protein: 5 g

168. Herbed Radish Sauté

Difficulty: Easy
Preparation Time: 5 minutes
Cooking Time: 15 minutes
Servings: 4
Ingredients:
- 2 bunches red radishes; halved
- 2 tbsp parsley; chopped.
- 1 tbsp balsamic vinegar
- 1 tbsp olive oil
- Salt and black pepper to taste.

Directions:
1. Take a bowl and mix the radishes with the remaining ingredients except for the parsley, toss and put them in your air fryer's basket.
2. Cook at 400°F for 15 minutes, divide between plates, sprinkle the parsley on top, and serve as a side dish.

Nutrition:
- Calories: 180
- Fat: 4 g
- Carbs: 3 g
- Protein: 5 g

169. Roasted Tomatoes

Difficulty: Easy
Preparation Time: 5 minutes
Cooking Time: 15 minutes
Servings: 4
Ingredients:
- 8 tomatoes; halved
- 1/2 cup Parmesan; grated
- 1 tbsp basil, chopped
- 1/2 tsp onion powder
- 1/2 tsp oregano, dried
- 1/2 tsp smoked paprika
- 1/2 tsp garlic powder
- Cooking spray

Directions:
1. Mix all the ingredients in a bowl, except the cooking spray and the Parmesan cheese.
2. Arrange the tomatoes in your air fryer's pan, sprinkle the Parmesan on top, and grease with cooking spray.
3. Cook at 370°F for 15 minutes, divide between plates and serve.

Nutrition:
- Calories: 200
- Fat: 7 g
- Carbs: 4 g
- Protein: 6 g

170. Kale and Walnuts

Difficulty: Easy
Preparation Time: 5 minutes
Cooking Time: 15 minutes
Servings: 4
Ingredients:
- ½ cup garlic cloves
- 10 cups kale; roughly chopped
- 1/3 cup Parmesan, grated
- 1/2 cup almond milk
- 1/4 cup walnuts; chopped
- 1 tbsp butter; melted
- 1/4 tsp nutmeg, ground
- Salt and black pepper to taste

Directions:
1. In a pan that fits into the air fryer, combine all the ingredients, toss, put the pan into the machine and cook at 360°F for 15 minutes.
2. Divide between plates and serve.

Nutrition:
- Calories: 160
- Fat: 7 g
- Carbs: 4 g
- Protein: 5 g

171. Bok Choy and Butter Sauce

Difficulty: Easy
Preparation Time: 5 minutes
Cooking Time: 15 minutes
Servings: 4
Ingredients:
- 3 bok choy heads; trimmed and cut into strips
- 1 tbsp butter, melted
- 2 tbsp chicken stock
- 1 tsp lemon juice
- 1 tbsp olive oil
- A pinch of salt and black pepper

Directions:
1. In a pan that fits into your air fryer, mix all the ingredients, toss, put the pan into the oven and cook at 380°F for 15 minutes.
2. Divide between plates and serve as a side dish.

Nutrition:
- Calories: 141
- Fat: 3 g
- Carbs: 4 g
- Protein: 3 g

172. Turmeric Mushroom

Difficulty: Easy
Preparation Time: 5 minutes
Cooking Time: 15 minutes
Servings: 4
Ingredients:
- 1 lb. brown mushrooms
- 2 garlic cloves; minced
- 1/4 tsp cinnamon powder
- 1 tsp olive oil
- 1/2 tsp turmeric powder
- Salt and black pepper to taste.

Directions:
1. In a bowl, combine all the ingredients and toss.
2. Put the mushrooms in your air fryer's basket and cook at 370°F for 15 minutes.
3. Divide the mix between plates and serve as a side dish.

Nutrition:
- Calories: 208
- Fat: 7 g
- Carbs: 5 g
- Protein: 7 g

173. Berry Mojito

Difficulty: Easy
Preparation Time: 10 minutes
Cooking Time: 0 minutes
Servings: 2
Ingredients:
- 2 tbsp fresh lime juice
- 6 fresh mint leaves
- 1 packet Mixed Berry Flavor Infuser
- 16 ounces seltzer water
- Ice cubes, as required

Directions:
1. In the bottom of 2 cocktail glasses, divide the lime juice and mint leaves.
2. With the bottom end of a spoon, gently muddle the mint leaves.
3. Now, divide the Berry Infuser and seltzer water into each glass and stir to combine.
4. Place ice cubes in each glass and serve.

Nutrition:
- Calories: 5
- Fat: 12.6 g
- Carbohydrates: 1.1 g
- Fiber: 0.5 g
- Sugar: 0 g
- Protein: 0 g
- Sodium: 0 mg

174. Coconut Smoothie

Difficulty: Easy
Preparation Time: 5 minutes
Cooking Time: 0 minutes
Servings: 1
Ingredients:
- 1 sachet Essential Creamy Vanilla Shake
- 6 ounces unsweetened almond milk
- 6 ounces of diet ginger ale
- 2 tbsp unsweetened coconut, shredded
- ¼ tsp rum extract
- ½ cup ice

Directions:
1. In a small blender, place all the ingredients and pulse until smooth.
2. Transfer the smoothie into a serving glass and serve immediately.

Nutrition:
- Calories: 120
- Fat: 6.2 g
- Carbohydrates: 15.9 g
- Fiber: 5.6 g
- Sugar: 7.6 g
- Protein: 15 g
- Sodium: 124 mg

175. Tiramisu Shake

Difficulty: Medium
Preparation Time: 5 minutes
Cooking Time: 0 minutes
Servings: 1
Ingredients:
- 1 packet cappuccino mix
- 1 tbsp sugar-free chocolate syrup
- ½ cup water
- ½ cup ice, crushed

Directions:
1. In a small blender, add all the ingredients and pulse until smooth and creamy.
2. Transfer the shake into a serving glass and serve immediately.

Nutrition:
- Calories: 107
- Fat: 0 g
- Carbohydrates: 15 g
- Fiber: 4.5 g
- Sugar: 8 g
- Protein: 14 g
- Sodium: 150 mg

176. Vanilla Shake

Difficulty: Easy
Preparation Time: 5 minutes
Cooking Time: 0 minutes
Servings: 1
Ingredients:
- ½ packet Vanilla Shake Fueling
- ½ packet Gingerbread Fueling
- ½ cup unsweetened almond milk
- ½ cup water
- 8 ice cubes

Directions:
1. In a small blender, place all the ingredients and pulse until smooth.
2. Transfer the shake into a serving glass and serve immediately.

Nutrition:
- Calories: 130
- Fat: 3.3 g
- Carbohydrates: 15 g
- Fiber: 4.5 g
- Sugar: 6 g
- Protein: 13 g
- Sodium: 100 mg

177. Shamrock Shake

Difficulty: Easy
Preparation Time: 5 minutes
Cooking Time: 0 minutes
Servings: 1
Ingredients:
- 1 packet Vanilla Shake
- 6 ounces unsweetened almond milk
- ¼ tsp peppermint extract
- 1–2 drops of green food coloring
- 1 cup ice cubes

Directions:
1. In a small blender, place all the ingredients and pulse until smooth.
2. Transfer the shake into a serving glass and serve immediately.

Nutrition:
- Calories: 120
- Fat: 3.9 g
- Carbohydrates: 13.5 g
- Fiber: 4.7 g
- Sugar: 6.1 g
- Protein: 11.7 g
- Sodium: 80 mg

178. Chocolate Shake

Difficulty: Easy
Preparation Time: 10 minutes
Cooking Time: 0 minutes
Servings: 1
Ingredients:
- 1 packet cappuccino mix
- ½ cup water
- 1 tbsp sugar-free chocolate syrup
- ½ cup ice, crushed

Directions:
1. In a small blender, place all the ingredients and pulse until smooth.

2. Transfer the shake into a serving glass and serve immediately.

Nutrition:
- Calories: 107
- Fat: 0.5 g
- Carbohydrates: 15 g
- Fiber: 4.5 g
- Sugar: 8 g
- Protein: 13 g
- Sodium: 121 mg

179. Peppermint Mocha

Difficulty: Easy
Preparation Time: 5 minutes
Cooking Time: 0 minutes
Servings: 1
Ingredients:
- 1 sachet Essential Velvety Hot Chocolate
- 6 ounces of freshly brewed coffee
- ¼ cup warm unsweetened almond milk
- ¼ tsp peppermint extract
- 1 tbsp whipped topping
- A pinch ground cinnamon

Directions:
1. In a serving mug, place the Hot Chocolate sachet, coffee, almond milk, and peppermint extract and stir until well blended.
2. Top the hot chocolate with whipped topping and sprinkle with cinnamon.
3. Serve immediately.

Nutrition:
- Calories: 133
- Fat: 1.1 g
- Carbohydrates: 15.2 g
- Fiber: 4.4 g
- Sugar: 10 g
- Protein: 14.6 g
- Sodium: 110 mg

180. Pumpkin Frappe

Difficulty: Easy
Preparation Time: 5 minutes
Cooking Time: 0 minutes
Servings: 1
Ingredients:
- 1 sachet Essential Spiced Gingerbread
- 4 ounces strong brewed coffee
- 4 ounces unsweetened almond milk
- 1/8 tsp pumpkin pie spice
- ½ cup ice
- 1 tbsp whipped topping

Directions:
1. In a blender, add the Spiced Gingerbread sachet, coffee, almond milk, pumpkin pie spice and ice, and pulse until smooth.
2. Transfer the mixture into a glass and top with whipped topping.
3. Serve immediately.

Nutrition:
- Calories: 138
- Fat: 4.8 g
- Carbohydrates: 16.4 g
- Fiber: 4.5 g
- Sugar: 5.3 g
- Protein: 11.7 g
- Sodium: 54 mg

181. Vanilla Frappe

Difficulty: Easy
Preparation Time: 5 minutes
Cooking Time: 0 minutes
Servings: 1
Ingredients:
- 1 sachet Essential Vanilla Shake
- 8 ounces unsweetened almond milk
- ½ cup ice
- 1 tbsp whipped topping

Directions:
1. In a blender, add the Vanilla Shake sachet, almond milk and ice, and pulse until smooth.
2. Transfer the mixture into a glass and top with whipped topping.

3. Serve immediately.

Nutrition:
- Calories: 155
- Fat: 4.5 g
- Carbohydrates: 15.2 g
- Fiber: 4.9 g
- Sugar: 7.2 g
- Protein: 42.3 g
- Sodium: 59 mg

182. Chocolate Frappe

Difficulty: Easy
Preparation Time: 5 minutes
Cooking Time: 0 minutes
Servings: 1
Ingredients:
- 1 sachet Essential Frosty Mint Chocolate Soft Serve Treat
- 4 ounces strong brewed coffee
- 4 ounces unsweetened almond milk
- 1½ tbsp sugar-free chocolate syrup, divided
- ¼ tsp peppermint extract
- ½ cup ice
- 1 tbsp whipped topping

Directions:
1. In a blender, add the Chocolate sachet, coffee, almond milk, 1 tbsp of chocolate syrup, peppermint extract and ice, and pulse until smooth.
2. Transfer the mixture into a glass and top with whipped topping.
3. Drizzle with the remaining chocolate syrup and serve immediately.

Nutrition:
- Calories: 148
- Fat: 4.8 g
- Carbohydrates: 18 g
- Fiber: 4.5 g
- Sugar: 7.2 g
- Protein: 11.7 g
- Sodium: 125 mg

183. Caramel Macchiato Frappe

Difficulty: Intermediate
Preparation Time: 10 minutes
Cooking Time: 0 minutes
Servings: 1
Ingredients:
- 8 ounces unsweetened cashew milk
- 1 sachet Essential Caramel Macchiato Shake
- ½ cup ice
- 2 tbsp whipped topping
- 1 tbsp sugar-free caramel syrup

Directions:
1. In a blender, add the Macchiato Shake sachet, cashew milk and ice, and pulse until smooth.
2. Transfer the mixture into a glass and top with whipped topping.
3. Drizzle with caramel syrup and serve immediately.

Nutrition:
- Calories: 139
- Fat: 4.1 g
- Carbohydrates: 16 g
- Fiber: 3 g
- Sugar: 8.5 g
- Protein: 11.2 g
- Sodium: 329 mg

184. Eggnog

Difficulty: Easy
Preparation Time: 10 minutes
Cooking Time: 0 minutes
Servings: 1
Ingredients:
- 1 sachet Essential Vanilla Shake
- 8 ounces unsweetened almond milk
- 1 egg (yolk and white separated)
- ¼ tsp rum extract
- Pinch ground nutmeg

Directions:
1. In a blender, add the Vanilla Shake sachet, almond milk and egg yolk, and pulse until smooth.

2. In the bowl of a stand mixer, place egg white and beat on medium speed until stiff peaks form.
3. Place the whipped egg whites into a serving glass and top with the shake mixture.
4. Stir the mixture and sprinkle with nutmeg.
5. Serve immediately.

Nutrition:
- Calories: 211
- Fat: 8.2 g
- Carbohydrates: 15.3 g
- Fiber: 5 g
- Sugar: 7.4 g
- Protein: 20.5 g
- Sodium: 100 mg

185. Pumpkin Spiced Latte

Difficulty: Easy
Preparation Time: 5 minutes
Cooking Time: 1 minute
Servings: 1
Ingredients:
- ½ cup unsweetened cashew milk
- 2 tbsp pumpkin puree
- ½ cup strong brewed coffee
- 1 sachet Essential Spiced Gingerbread

Directions:
1. In a microwave-safe mug, place cashew milk and pumpkin puree and microwave for 1 minute.
2. Remove from microwave and immediately stir in coffee and Gingerbread sachet until smooth.
3. Serve immediately.

Nutrition:
- Calories: 134
- Fat: 3.1 g
- Carbohydrates: 14 g
- Fiber: 4.9 g
- Sugar: 6 g
- Protein: 11.5 g
- Sodium: 264 mg

186. Hot Chocolate

Difficulty: Easy
Preparation Time: 10 minutes
Cooking Time: 2 minutes
Servings: 1
Ingredients:
- 1 sachet Essential Velvety Hot Chocolate
- ½ tsp ground cinnamon
- A pinch cayenne pepper
- 6 ounces unsweetened almond milk
- 1 tbsp whipped cream

Directions:
1. In a serving mug, place all the ingredients except for whipped cream and beat until well blended.
2. Microwave on high for about 2 minutes.
3. Top with whipped cream and serve.

Nutrition:
- Calories: 185
- Fat: 7.6 g
- Carbohydrates: 15.9 g
- Fiber: 5.3 g
- Sugar: 10 g
- Protein: 15.1 g
- Sodium: 80 mg

187. Cherry Mocha Popsicles

Difficulty: Easy
Preparation Time: 10 minutes
Cooking Time: 45 seconds
Servings: 6
Ingredients:
- 1 cup unsweetened almond milk
- 3 sachets Dark Chocolate Covered Cherry Shake
- 1 tsp vanilla extract
- 1 tbsp instant espresso powder
- 2 cups plain low-fat Greek yogurt
- 1–2 packets zero-calorie sugar substitute

Directions:
1. In a microwave-safe mug, place the almond milk and microwave on High for about 45 seconds.

2. Remove the mug from the microwave and immediately stir in the espresso powder until dissolved completely.
3. Set aside to cool completely.
4. In a blender, add the cooled espresso milk and remaining ingredients and pulse until smooth.
5. Divide the mixture into 6 large Popsicle molds and freeze overnight.

Nutrition:
- Calories: 104
- Fat: 5.2 g
- Carbohydrates: 13.7 g
- Fiber: 2.2 g
- Sugar: 8.4 g
- Protein: 10.4 g
- Sodium: 90 mg

188. Yogurt Cookie Dough

Difficulty: Easy
Preparation Time: 5 minutes
Cooking Time: 0 minutes
Servings: 1
Ingredients:
- 1 sachet Essential Chocolate Chip Cookie
- 1 (5.3-ounce) container low-fat plain Greek yogurt

Directions:
1. In a bowl add Chocolate Chip Cookie and yogurt and mix until well combined.
2. Refrigerate to chill before serving.

Nutrition:
- Calories: 197
- Fat: 3.6 g
- Carbohydrates: 22 g
- Fiber: 4 g
- Sugar: 15 g
- Protein: 18.5 g
- Sodium: 345 mg

189. Chocolate Coconut Pie

Difficulty: Easy
Preparation Time: 10 minutes
Cooking Time: 20 seconds
Servings: 2
Ingredients:
- 1 sachet Drizzled Chocolate Fudge Crisp Bar
- Olive oil cooking spray
- 2 tbsp whipped topping
- 1 sachet Essential Chocolate Fudge Pudding
- ½ cup unsweetened coconut milk
- 1 tbsp unsweetened coconut, shredded

Directions:
1. In a microwave-safe bowl, add the Chocolate bar and microwave on High for about 15–20 seconds.
2. Place the melted bar into a lightly greased ramekin and with the back of a spoon, press it slightly.
3. In a bowl, add the Fudge pudding and milk and mix well.
4. Place the pudding mixture over the bar in the ramekin and refrigerate for about 30 minutes.
5. Top with whipped topping and coconut and serve.

Nutrition:
- Calories: 265
- Fat: 18.8 g
- Carbohydrates: 16.1 g
- Fiber: 5.1 g
- Sugar: 6.4 g
- Protein: 12.6 g
- Sodium: 163 mg

190. Caramel Crunch Parfait

Difficulty: Easy
Preparation Time: 10 minutes
Cooking Time: 0 minutes
Servings: 1
Ingredients:
- 6 ounces low-fat plain Greek yogurt
- ½ packet stevia
- ¼ tsp vanilla extract
- 2 tbsp whipped topping
- 1 sachet Puffed Sweet & Salty Snacks, crushed
- 1 tbsp sugar-free caramel syrup

Directions:
1. In a bowl, mix the yogurt, stevia, and vanilla extract.
2. Top with whipped topping Puffed Snack sachet.
3. Drizzle with caramel syrup and serve.

Nutrition:
- Calories: 150
- Fat: 6.2 g
- Carbohydrates: 16.9 g
- Fiber: 1 g
- Sugar: 7.9 g
- Protein: 7.4 g
- Sodium: 151 mg

191. <u>Chocolate Berry Parfait</u>

Difficulty: Easy
Preparation Time: 10 minutes
Cooking Time: 0 minutes
Servings: 2
Ingredients:
- 1 sachet Chocolate Cherry Ganache Bar
- 1½ cups low-fat plain Greek yogurt
- ¼ cup strawberry-flavored light cream cheese, softened
- 1 tbsp unsweetened cocoa powder
- 1–2 packets zero-calorie sugar substitute
- 2/3-ounce almonds, sliced

Directions:
1. In a blender, add all the ingredients and pulse until desired consistency is achieved.
2. Serve immediately.

Nutrition:
- Calories: 311
- Fat: 18.6 g
- Carbohydrates: 23 g
- Fiber: 4.1 g
- Sugar: 16 g
- Protein: 15.2 g
- Sodium: 263 mg

192. <u>Brownie Pudding</u>

Difficulty: Easy
Preparation Time: 5 minutes
Cooking Time: 0 minutes
Servings: 1
Ingredients:
- 1 (5.3-ounce) container low-fat plain Greek yogurt
- 1 sachet Brownie Mix

Directions:
1. In a bowl, add yogurt and Brownie Mix sachet and mix well.
2. Refrigerate to chill before serving.

Nutrition:
- Calories: 190
- Fat: 2 g
- Carbohydrates: 20 g
- Fiber: 4 g
- Sugar: 13 g
- Protein: 24.7 g
- Sodium: 223 mg

193. <u>Brownie Peanut Butter Pudding</u>

Difficulty: Easy
Preparation Time: 5 minutes
Cooking Time: 0 minutes
Servings: 1
Ingredients:
- 1 packet Brownie
- 1 (5.3-ounce) container low-fat plain Greek yogurt
- 1 tbsp peanut butter powder
- A dash vanilla extract

Directions:
1. In a bowl add all the ingredients and mix until well combined.
2. Refrigerate to chill before serving.

Nutrition:
- Calories: 215
- Fat: 2.7 g
- Carbohydrates: 22 g
- Fiber: 4.7 g
- Sugar: 14.4 g

- Protein: 27.4 g
- Sodium: 225 mg

194. Chia Seed Pudding

Difficulty: Easy
Preparation Time: 10 minutes
Cooking Time: 0 minutes
Servings: 1
Ingredients:
- 2 sachets Chia Bliss Smoothie
- 1 cup unsweetened almond milk
- ¼ cup chia seeds

Directions:
1. In a serving bowl, add all the ingredients and mix until well blended.
2. Refrigerate overnight before serving.

Nutrition:
- Calories: 188
- Fat: 17.8 g
- Carbohydrates: 20 g
- Fiber: 9 g
- Sugar: 6 g
- Protein: 14.5 g
- Sodium: 90 mg

195. Chocolate Cake Fries

Difficulty: Medium
Preparation Time: 10 minutes
Cooking Time: 4 minutes
Servings: 2
Ingredients:
- 2 sachets essential Golden Chocolate Chip Pancakes
- ¼ cup liquid egg substitute
- 2 tsp vegetable oil

Directions:
1. In a bowl, add Pancakes sachets and egg substitute and mix until well combined.
2. Place the mixture into a resealable plastic bag.
3. Cut off a small hole on top of the bag.
4. In a skillet, heat oil over medium heat.
5. In the skillet, pipe the mixture in long, straight lines and cook for about 2 minutes per side.
6. Serve warm.

Nutrition:
- Calories: 167
- Fat: 6 g
- Carbohydrates: 11 g
- Fiber: 4 g
- Sugar: 4.2 g
- Protein: 14.8 g
- Sodium: 304 mg

196. French Toast Sticks

Difficulty: Easy
Preparation Time: 15 minutes
Cooking Time: 4 minutes
Servings: 3
Ingredients:
- 2 sachets Essential Cinnamon Crunchy Oat Cereal
- 6 tbsp egg liquid substitute
- 2 tbsp low-fat cream cheese, softened
- Olive oil cooking spray

Directions:
1. In a food processor, add the cereal sachets and pulse until fine-breadcrumbs-like consistency is achieved.
2. Add the egg liquid substitute and cream cheese and pulse until a dough forms.
3. Divide the dough into 6 portions and shape each into a breadstick.
4. Heat a lightly greased skillet over medium-high heat and cook the French toast sticks for about 2 minutes per side or until golden brown.
5. Serve warm.

Nutrition:
- Calories: 107
- Fat: 3 g
- Carbohydrates: 10.3 g
- Fiber: 2.6 g
- Sugar: 1.5 g
- Protein: 11.6 g
- Sodium: 164 mg

197. Fudge Balls

Difficulty: Easy
Preparation Time: 10 minutes
Cooking Time: 0 minutes
Servings: 2
Ingredients:
- 1 sachet chocolate pudding
- 1 sachet chocolate shake
- 4 tbsp peanut butter powder
- ¼ cup unsweetened almond milk
- 2 tbsp water

Directions:
1. In a small bowl, add all the ingredients and mix until well combined.
2. Make 8 small equal-sized balls from the mixture.
3. Arrange the balls onto a parchment paper-lined baking sheet and refrigerate until set before serving.

Nutrition:
- Calories: 218
- Fat: 5.3 g
- Carbohydrates: 15.3 g
- Fiber: 8.3 g
- Sugar: 7 g
- Protein: 30 g
- Sodium: 111 mg

198. Peanut Butter Bites

Difficulty: Easy
Preparation Time: 10 minutes
Cooking Time: 1 minute
Servings: 1
Ingredients:
- 2 tbsp peanut butter powder
- 1 tbsp water
- 1 sachet Essential Creamy Double Peanut Butter Crisp Bar

Directions:
1. In a bowl, add the peanut butter powder and water and mix until a smooth paste is formed.
2. On a microwave-safe plate, place the Crisp Bar and microwave for about 15 seconds or until soft.
3. Add the warm bar pieces into the bowl of water mixture and mix until a dough forms.
4. Make small 4 equal-sized balls from the dough and arrange them onto a parchment paper-lined plate.
5. Refrigerate until set before serving.

Nutrition:
- Calories: 190
- Fat: 5.5 g
- Carbohydrates: 17 g
- Fiber: 4 g
- Sugar: 9 g
- Protein: 17 g
- Sodium: 300 mg

199. Yogurt Cereal Bark

Difficulty: Easy
Preparation Time: 10 minutes
Cooking Time: 0 minutes
Servings: 2
Ingredients:
- 12 ounces low-fat plain Greek yogurt
- 1–2 packets zero-calorie sugar substitute
- 1 sachet Essential Red Berry Crunch O's Cereal

Directions:
1. Line an 8x8-inch baking dish with a piece of foil.
2. In a bowl, add yogurt and sugar substitute and mix well.
3. Place the yogurt mixture into the prepared baking dish and spread in an even layer.
4. Sprinkle the Cereal sachet on top evenly.
5. Freeze overnight or until the bark is hard.
6. With a sharp knife, cut the bark into small pieces and serve.

Nutrition:
- Calories: 157
- Fat: 2.8 g
- Carbohydrates: 19.5 g
- Fiber: 2 g
- Sugar: 8.5 g

- Protein: 13 g
- Sodium: 150 mg

200. Chocolate Crunch Cookies

Difficulty: Intermediate
Preparation Time: 10 minutes
Cooking Time: 2 minutes 20 seconds
Servings: 2
Ingredients:
- 1 sachet Brownie Mix
- 1 Peanut Butter Chocolate Crunch Bar
- 3 tbsp water

Directions:
1. In a bowl, add the brownie mix and water and mix well. Set aside.
2. In a microwave-safe bowl, place the crunch bar and microwave on High for about 20 seconds or until it is slightly melted.
3. Add the crunch bar into the brownie mixture and mix until well combined.
4. Divide the mixture into 2 greased ramekins and microwave on High for about 2 minutes.
5. Remove from microwave and set aside to cool for about 5 minutes before serving.

Nutrition:
- Calories: 110
- Fat: 3 g
- Carbohydrates: 13.5 g
- Fiber: 4 g
- Sugar: 6 g
- Protein: 11 g
- Sodium: 165 mg

201. Oatmeal Cookies

Difficulty: Easy
Preparation Time: 10 minutes
Cooking Time: 15 minutes
Servings: 2
Ingredients:
1 oatmeal raisin crunch bar
1 packet oatmeal
1/8 tsp ground cinnamon
1 packet stevia powder
1/8 tsp baking powder
½ tsp vanilla extract
1/3 cup water

Directions:
1. Preheat your oven to 350°F. Line a cookie sheet with parchment paper.
2. In a microwave-safe bowl, place the crunch bar and microwave on High for about 15 seconds or until it is slightly melted.
3. In the bowl with the crunch bar, add the remaining ingredients and mix until well combined.
4. Set the mixture aside for about 5 minutes.
5. With a spoon, place 4 cookies onto the prepared cookie sheet in a single layer and with your fingers, press each ball slightly.
6. Bake for approximately 12–15 minutes or until golden brown.
7. Remove from the oven and place the cookie sheet onto a wire rack to cool for about 5 minutes.
8. Now, invert the cookies onto the wire rack to cool before serving.

Nutrition:
- Calories: 114
- Fat: 2.3 g
- Carbohydrates: 14.4 g
- Fiber: 4.1 g
- Sugar: 3.1 g
- Protein: 11 g
- Sodium: 147 mg

202. Peanut Butter Cookies

Difficulty: Easy
Preparation Time: 10 minutes
Cooking Time: 12 minutes
Servings: 4
Ingredients:
- 4 sachets Essential Silky Peanut Butter Shake
- ¼ tsp baking powder
- ¼ cup unsweetened almond milk
- 1 tbsp margarine, softened
- ¼ tsp vanilla extract
- 1/8 tsp sea salt

Directions:
1. Preheat your oven to 350°F. Line a cookie sheet with parchment paper.
2. In a bowl, add the Peanut Butter Shake and baking powder and mix well.
3. Add the almond milk, margarine and vanilla extract, and mix until well blended.
4. With a spoon, place 8 cookies onto the prepared cookie sheet in a single layer and with a fork, press each ball slightly.
5. Sprinkle each cookie with salt.
6. Bake for approximately 10–12 minutes.
7. Remove from the oven and place the cookie sheet onto a wire rack to cool for about 5 minutes.
8. Now, invert the cookies onto the wire rack to cool before serving.

Nutrition:
- Calories: 57
- Fat: 3.4 g
- Carbohydrates: 4 g
- Fiber: 0.1 g
- Sugar: 0.2 g
- Protein: 2.8 g
- Sodium: 22 mg

203. Mint Cookies

Difficulty: Medium
Preparation Time: 15 minutes
Cooking Time: 10 minutes
Servings: 4
Ingredients:
- 2 sachet Essential Chocolate Mint Cookie Bars
- 2 sachet Essential Decadent Double Chocolate Brownie
- 2 tbsp unsweetened almond milk
- 2 egg whites

Directions:
1. Preheat your oven to 350°F.
2. Line a cookie sheet with parchment paper.
3. In a food processor, add the Chocolate Bars and pulse until crushed.
4. Transfer the crushed bar into a bowl with the remaining ingredients and mix until well blended.
5. With a spoon, place 8 cookies onto the prepared cookie sheet in a single layer, and with your fingers, press each ball slightly.
6. Bake for approximately 13–15 minutes.
7. Remove from the oven and place the cookie sheet onto a wire rack to cool for about 5 minutes.
8. Now, invert the cookies onto the wire rack to cool before serving.

Nutrition:
- Calories: 120
- Fat: 2.8 g
- Carbohydrates: 14.2 g
- Fiber: 4 g
- Sugar: 16 g
- Protein: 12.8 g
- Sodium: 90 mg

204. Gingersnap Cookies

Difficulty: Easy
Preparation Time: 10 minutes
Cooking Time: 20 minutes
Servings: 1
Ingredients:
- 1 sachet Essential Spiced Gingerbread
- 2 tbsp cold water
- Olive oil cooking spray
- 2 tbsp low-fat whipped cream cheese spread
- 1/8 tsp vanilla tract
- 3–5 drops liquid stevia

Directions:
1. Preheat your oven to 350°F.
2. Lightly grease a cookie sheet.
3. In a bowl, add the Spiced Gingerbread sachet and beat until smooth.
4. With a small spoon, place about 3 cookies onto the prepared cookie sheet in a single layer.
5. Bake for approximately 18–20 minutes or until golden brown.
6. Remove from the oven and place the cookie sheet onto a wire rack to cool for about 5 minutes.
7. Now, invert the cookies onto the wire rack to cool before serving.

8. Meanwhile, in a small bowl, place cream cheese, vanilla extract, and stevia and beat until smooth.
9. Spread frosting over cookies and serve.

Nutrition:
- Calories: 262
- Fat: 12.6 g
- Carbohydrates: 19.1 g
- Fiber: 5 g
- Sugar: 6.1 g
- Protein: 12 g
- Sodium: 270 mg

205. Crunch Sandwich Cookies

Difficulty: Easy
Preparation Time: 10 minutes
Cooking Time: 15 seconds
Servings: 1
Ingredients:
- 1 packet S'more Crunch Bar
- 1 tbsp whipped topping

Directions:
1. Line 2 cups of a muffin tin with cupcake liners.
2. Break the Crunch Bar into 2 pieces.
3. In a microwave-safe bowl, place the bar pieces and microwave for about 15 seconds.
4. Place the bar into the prepared muffin cups evenly and with your fingers press down to form round cookies.
5. Freeze for about 15 minutes.
6. Remove from the freezer and place the cookies onto a plate.
7. Spread whipped topping between both cookies and serve.

Nutrition:
- Calories: 118
- Fat: 3.2 g
- Carbohydrates: 13.4 g
- Fiber: 4 g
- Sugar: 6.2 g
- Protein: 11.1 g
- Sodium: 174 mg

206. Sandwich Cookies

Difficulty: Easy
Preparation Time: 10 minutes
Cooking Time: 12 minutes
Servings: 1
Ingredients:
- 1 sachet Chocolate Chip Soft Bake
- 1/8 tsp baking powder
- 3 tbsp water
- 1 tbsp whipped cream

Directions:
1. Preheat your oven to 375°F. Line a cookie sheet with parchment paper.
2. In a bowl, mix the Chocolate Bake sachet and baking powder.
3. Slowly, add the water and mix until well blended.
4. Divide the dough into 2 pieces and place it onto the prepared cookie sheet.
5. With your hands, press each dough piece into a cookie shape.
6. Bake for approximately 12 minutes.
7. Remove from the oven and place the cookie sheet onto a wire rack to cool for about 5 minutes.
8. Now, invert the cookies onto the wire rack to cool before serving.
9. Arrange a cookie, smooth side upwards.
10. Place the whipped cream on top of the cookie.
11. Cover with the remaining cookie and lightly press together.
12. Serve.

Nutrition:
- Calories: 154
- Fat: 6.6 g
- Carbohydrates: 15.7 g
- Fiber: 4 g
- Sugar: 7 g
- Protein: 11.3 g
- Sodium: 120 mg

207. Snickerdoodles

Difficulty: Easy
Preparation Time: 10 minutes
Cooking Time: 8 minutes
Servings: 2
Ingredients:

- 2 packets French Vanilla Shake
- 1 packet Splenda with Fiber
- 1 tsp baking powder
- ¼ tsp ground cinnamon
- 1 tsp vanilla extract
- ¼ cup water

Directions:
1. Preheat your oven to 350°F. Line a cookie sheet with parchment paper.
2. In a bowl, add the Vanilla Shake packet, Splenda, baking powder, and cinnamon and mix well.
3. Add the vanilla extract and mix well.
4. Slowly, add the water and mix until a paste is formed.
5. With a spoon, place 4 cookies onto the prepared cookie sheet in a single layer, and with your fingers, press each ball slightly.
6. Bake for approximately 8 minutes.
7. Remove from the oven and place the cookie sheet onto a wire rack to cool for about 5 minutes.
8. Now, invert the cookies onto the wire rack to cool before serving.

Nutrition:

- Calories: 74
- Fat: 0.2 g
- Carbohydrates: 10.2 g
- Fiber: 2.2 g
- Sugar: 5.8 g
- Protein: 7 g
- Sodium: 111 mg

208. Chocolate Whoopie Pies

Difficulty: Easy
Preparation Time: 20 minutes
Cooking Time: 15 minutes
Servings: 2
Ingredients:

- 2 sachets Decadent Double Chocolate Brownie
- ¼ tsp baking powder
- 6 tbsp unsweetened almond milk, divided
- 3 tbsp egg liquid substitute
- 1 tsp vegetable oil
- ¼ cup powdered peanut butter

Directions:
1. Preheat your oven to 350°F. Grease 4 cups of a muffin tin.
2. In a small bowl, add the Chocolate Brownie, ¼ cup of almond milk, egg substitute and oil, and mix until well blended.
3. Place the mixture into the prepared muffin cups.
4. Bake for approximately 18–20 minutes or until a toothpick inserted in the center comes out clean.
5. Remove the muffin tin from the oven and place it onto a wire rack to cool for about 10 minutes.
6. Carefully invert the muffins onto the wire rack to cool completely.
7. Meanwhile, in a bowl, add the remaining almond milk and peanut butter and mix well.
8. After cooling, slice each muffin in half horizontally.
9. Spread the peanut butter powder mixture over the bottom half of each muffin.
10. Cover each bottom half with the remaining muffin halves and serve.

Nutrition:

- Calories: 141
- Fat: 5.4 g
- Carbohydrates: 13.3 g
- Fiber: 4.2 g
- Sugar: 5.2 g
- Protein: 13.6 g
- Sodium: 120 mg

209. Brownie Bites

Difficulty: Medium
Preparation Time: 10 minutes
Cooking Time: 0 minutes
Servings: 6
Ingredients:
- 3 tbsp peanut butter powder
- 1 cup plus 3 tbsp water, divided
- 6 sachets Double Chocolate Brownie Mix
- 1 cup water

Directions:
1. In a small bowl, add the peanut butter powder and 3 tbsp of water and mix until well combined.
2. In another bowl, add Double Chocolate Brownie sachets and the remaining water and mix until well combined.
3. In the bottom of 6 silicone molds, place the peanut butter powder mixture evenly and top with the brownie mixture.
4. Freeze the molds until set completely.
5. Remove from the freezer and set aside for about 30–40 minutes before serving.

Nutrition:
- Calories: 137
- Fat: 3 g
- Carbohydrates: 16 g
- Fiber: 5.1 g
- Sugar: 8 g
- Protein: 15 g
- Sodium: 270 mg

210. Chocolate Haystacks

Difficulty: Easy
Preparation Time: 10 minutes
Cooking Time: 0 minutes
Servings: 1
Ingredients:
- 1 sachet Brownie Mix
- 3 tbsp water
- 1 tbsp peanut butter powder
- 1 packet stevia powder
- 1 packet Cinnamon Pretzel Sticks, crushed

Directions:
1. In a small bowl, add the brownie mix and water and mix until a paste forms.
2. Add peanut butter powder and stevia and mix until well combined.
3. Add the crushed pretzels and mix until well combined.
4. With a spoon, place 6 haystacks onto a piece of foil and freeze for about 1 hour or until set.

Nutrition:
- Calories: 127
- Fat: 3.1 g
- Carbohydrates: 15.5 g
- Fiber: 5 g
- Sugar: 4.5 g
- Protein: 15 g
- Sodium: 141 mg

BREAKFAST RECIPES

211. Gluten-Free Pancakes

Difficulty: Easy
Preparation Time: 5 minutes
Cooking Time: 2 minutes
Servings: 2
Ingredients:
- 6 eggs
- 1 cup low-fat cream cheese
- 1 1/12 tsp baking powder
- 1 scoop protein powder
- 1/4 cup almond meal
- ¼ tsp salt

Directions:
1. Combine dry ingredients in a food processor. Add the eggs one after another and then the cream cheese. Mix it well.
2. Lightly grease a skillet with cooking spray and place over medium-high heat.
3. Pour the batter into the pan. Turn the pan gently to create round pancakes.
4. Cook for about 2 minutes on each side.
5. Serve pancakes with your favorite topping.

Nutrition:
- Dietary Fiber: 1 g
- Net Carbs: 5 g
- Protein: 25 g
- Total Fat: 14 g
- Calories: 288

212. Mushroom & Spinach Omelet

Difficulty: Easy
Preparation Time: 20 minutes
Cooking Time: 20 minutes
Servings: 3
Ingredients:
- 2 tbsp butter, divided
- 6–8 fresh mushrooms, sliced, 5 ounces
- Chives, chopped, optional
- Salt and pepper, to taste
- 1 handful baby spinach, about 1/2 ounce
- A pinch garlic powder
- 4 eggs, beaten
- 1-ounce shredded Swiss cheese

Directions:
1. In a very large saucepan, sauté the mushrooms in one tbsp of butter until soft. Season with salt, pepper, and garlic.
2. Remove the mushrooms from the pan and keep them warm. Heat the remaining tbsp of butter in the same skillet over medium heat.
3. Beat the eggs with a little salt and pepper and add to the hot butter. Turn the pan over to coat the entire bottom of the pan with egg. Once the egg is almost out, place the cheese over the middle of the tortilla.
4. Fill the cheese with spinach leaves and hot mushrooms. Let cook for about a minute for the spinach to start to wilt. Fold the empty side of the tortilla carefully over the filling and slide it onto a plate and sprinkle with chives, if desired.
5. Alternatively, you can make two tortillas using half the mushroom, spinach, and cheese filling in each.

Nutrition:
- Calories: 321
- Fat: 26 g
- Protein: 19 g
- Carbohydrate: 4 g
- Dietary Fiber: 1 g

213. Pizza Hack

Difficulty: Easy
Preparation Time: 5–10 minutes
Cooking Time: 15–20 minutes
Servings: 1
Ingredients:
- 1/4 fueling garlic mashed potato
- 1/2 egg whites
- 1/4 tbsp baking powder
- 3/4 oz. reduced-fat shredded mozzarella

- 1/8 cup sliced white mushrooms
- 1/16 cup pizza sauce
- 3/4 oz. ground beef
- 1/4 sliced black olives
- You also need a sauté pan, baking sheets, and parchment paper

Directions:
1. Start by preheating the oven to 400°F.
2. Mix your baking powder and garlic potato packet.
3. Add egg whites to your mixture and stir well until it blends.
4. Line the baking sheet with parchment paper and pour the mixed batter onto it.
5. Put another parchment paper on top of the batter and spread out the batter to a 1/8-inch circle.
6. Then place another baking sheet on top; this way, the batter is between two baking sheets.
7. Place into an oven and bake for about 8 minutes until the pizza crust is golden brown.
8. For the toppings, place your ground beef in a sauté pan and fry till it's brown, and wash your mushrooms very well.
9. After the crust is baked, remove the top layer of parchment paper carefully to prevent the foam from sticking to the pizza crust.
10. Put your toppings on top of the crust and bake for an extra 8 minutes.
11. Once ready, slide the pizza off the parchment paper and onto a plate.

Nutrition:
- Calories: 478
- Protein: 30 g
- Carbohydrates: 22 g
- Fats: 29 g

214. **Sweet Cashew Cheese Spread**

Difficulty: Easy
Preparation Time: 5 minutes
Cooking Time: 5 minutes
Servings: 10 servings
Ingredients:
- 5 drops Stevia
- 2 cups, raw Cashews
- 1/2 cup Water

Directions:
1. Soak the cashews overnight in water.
2. Next, drain the excess water then transfer cashews to a food processor.
3. Add in the stevia and the water.
4. Process until smooth.
5. Serve chilled. Enjoy.

Nutrition:
- Fat: 7 g
- Cholesterol: 0 mg
- Sodium: 12.6 mg
- Carbohydrates: 5.7 g

215. **Mini Zucchini Bites**

Difficulty: Easy
Preparation Time: 10 minutes
Cooking Time: 10 minutes
Servings: 6
Ingredients:
- 1 zucchini, cut into thick circles
- 3 cherry tomatoes, halved
- 1/2 cup parmesan cheese, grated
- Salt and pepper to taste
- 1 tsp chives, chopped

Directions:
1. Preheat the oven to 390°F.
2. Add wax paper to a baking sheet.
3. Arrange the zucchini pieces.
4. Add the cherry halves to each zucchini slice.
5. Add parmesan cheese, chives and sprinkle with salt and pepper.
6. Bake for 10 minutes.
7. Serve.

Nutrition:
- Fat: 1.0 g
- Cholesterol: 5.0 mg
- Sodium: 400.3 mg
- Potassium: 50.5 mg
- Carbohydrates: 7.3 g

216. Whole-Wheat Blueberry Muffins

Difficulty: Intermediate
Preparation Time: 5 minutes
Cooking Time: 25 minutes
Servings: 8
Ingredients:
- 1/2 cup plant-based milk
- 1/2 cup unsweetened applesauce
- 1/2 cup maple syrup
- 1 tsp vanilla extract
- 2 cups whole-wheat flour
- 1/2 tsp baking soda
- 1 cup blueberries

Directions:
1. Preheat the oven to 375°F.
2. In a large bowl, mix the milk, applesauce, maple syrup, and vanilla.
3. Stir in the flour and baking soda until no dry flour is left, and the batter is smooth.
4. Gently fold in the blueberries until they are evenly distributed throughout the batter.
5. In a muffin tin, fill eight muffin cups with three-quarters full of batter.
6. Bake for 25 minutes, or until you can stick a knife into the center of a muffin and it comes out clean. Allow cooling before serving.

Tip: both frozen and fresh blueberries will work great in this recipe. The only difference will be that muffins using fresh blueberries will cook slightly quicker than those using frozen.

Nutrition:
- Fat: 1 g
- Carbohydrates: 45 g
- Fiber: 2 g
- Protein: 4 g

217. Hemp Seed Porridge

Difficulty: Easy
Preparation Time: 5 minutes
Cooking Time: 5 minutes
Servings: 6
Ingredients:
- 3 cups cooked hemp seed
- 1 packet Stevia
- 1 cup coconut milk

Directions:
1. In a saucepan, mix the rice and the coconut milk over moderate heat for about 5 minutes as you stir it constantly.
2. Remove the pan from the burner then add the Stevia. Stir.
3. Serve in 6 bowls.
4. Enjoy.

Nutrition:
- Calories: 236 kcal
- Fat: 1.8 g
- Carbs: 48.3 g
- Protein: 7 g

218. Walnut Crunch Banana Bread

Difficulty: Medium
Preparation Time: 5 minutes
Cooking Time: 1 hour and 30 minutes
Servings: 1
Ingredients:
- 4 ripe bananas
- 1/4 cup maple syrup
- 1 tbsp apple cider vinegar
- 1 tsp vanilla extract
- 1 1/2 cups whole-wheat flour
- 1/2 tsp ground cinnamon
- 1/2 tsp baking soda
- 1/4 cup walnut pieces (optional)

Directions:
1. Preheat the oven to 350°F.
2. In a large bowl, use a fork or mixing spoon to mash the bananas until they reach a puréed consistency (small bits of banana are acceptable). Stir in the maple syrup, apple cider vinegar, and vanilla.
3. Stir in the flour, cinnamon, and baking soda. Fold in the walnut pieces (if using).
4. Gently pour the batter into a loaf pan, filling it no more than three-quarters of the way full. Bake for 1 hour, or until you can stick a knife into the middle and it comes out clean.

5. Remove from the oven and allow cooling on the countertop for a minimum of 30 minutes before serving.

Nutrition:
- Fat: 1g
- Carbohydrates: 40 g
- Fiber: 5 g
- Protein: 4 g

219. Plant-Powered Pancakes

Difficulty: Easy
Preparation Time: 5 minutes
Cooking Time: 15 minutes
Servings: 8
Ingredients:
- 1 cup whole-wheat flour
- 1 tsp baking powder
- 1/2 tsp ground cinnamon
- 1 cup plant-based milk
- 1/2 cup unsweetened applesauce
- 1/4 cup maple syrup
- 1 tsp vanilla extract

Directions:
1. In a large bowl, combine the flour, baking powder, and cinnamon.
2. Stir in the milk, applesauce, maple syrup, and vanilla until no dry flour is left, and the batter is smooth.
3. Heat a large, nonstick skillet or griddle over medium heat. For each pancake, pour 1/4 cup of batter onto the hot skillet. Once bubbles form over the top of the pancake and the sides begin to brown, flip and cook for 1 or 2 minutes more.
4. Repeat until all of the batter is used, and serve.

Nutrition:
- Fat: 2 g
- Carbohydrates: 44 g
- Fiber: 5 g
- Protein: 5 g

220. Mini Mac in a Bowl

Difficulty: Medium
Preparation Time: 5 minutes
Cooking Time: 15 minutes
Servings: 1
Ingredients:
- 5 ounces lean ground beef
- 2 tbsp diced white or yellow onion.
- 1/8 tsp onion powder
- 1/8 tsp white vinegar
- 1-ounce dill pickle slices
- 1 tsp sesame seed
- 3 cups shredded Romaine lettuce
- Cooking spray
- 2 tbsp reduced-fat shredded cheddar cheese
- 2 tbsp Bone light thousand islands as dressing

Directions:
1. Place a lightly greased small skillet on fire to heat.
2. Add your onion to cook for about 2-3 minutes.
3. Next, add the beef and allow cooking until it's brown.
4. Next, mix your vinegar and onion powder with the dressing.
5. Finally, top the lettuce with the cooked meat and sprinkle cheese on it, add your pickle slices.
6. Drizzle the mixture with the sauce and sprinkle the sesame seeds.
7. Your mini mac in a bowl is ready for consumption.

Nutrition:
- Calories: 150
- Protein: 21 g
- Carbohydrates: 32 g
- Fats: 19 g

221. Shake Cake Fueling

Difficulty: Easy
Preparation Time: 5 minutes
Cooking Time: 0 minutes
Servings: 1
Ingredients:
- 1 packet shakes.
- 1/4 tsp baking powder
- 2 tbsp eggbeaters or egg whites
- 2 tbsp water
- Other options that are not compulsory include sweeteners, reduced-fat cream cheese, etc.

Directions:
1. Begin by preheating the oven.
2. Mix all the ingredients. Begin with the dry ingredients, and then add the wet ingredients.
3. After the mixture/batter is ready, pour gently into muffin cups.
4. Inside the oven, place, and bake for about 16–18 minutes or until it is baked and ready. Allow it to cool completely.
5. Add additional toppings of your choice and ensure your delicious shake cake is refreshing.

Nutrition:
- Calories: 896
- Fat: 37 g
- Carbohydrate: 115 g
- Protein: 34 g

222. Biscuit Pizza

Difficulty: Easy
Preparation Time: 5 minutes
Cooking Time: 15–20 minutes
Servings: 1
Ingredients:
- 1/4 sachet buttermilk cheddar and herb biscuit
- 1/4 tbsp tomato sauce
- 1/4 tbsp low-fat shredded cheese
- ¼ bottle water
- Parchment paper

Directions:
1. Begin by preheating the oven to about 350°F
2. Mix the biscuit and water and stir properly.
3. In the parchment paper, pour the mixture and spread it into a thin circle. Allow cooking for 10 minutes.
4. Take it out and add the tomato sauce and shredded cheese.
5. Bake it for a few more minutes.

Nutrition:
- Calories: 478
- Protein: 30 g
- Carbohydrates: 22 g
- Fats: 29 g

223. Lean and Green Smoothie 1

Difficulty: Easy
Preparation Time: 5 minutes
Cooking Time: 0 minutes
Servings: 1
Ingredients:
- 2 1/2 cups kale leaves
- 3/4 cup chilled apple juice
- 1 cup cubed pineapple
- 1/2 cup frozen green grapes
- 1/2 cup chopped apple

Directions:
1. Place the pineapple, apple juice, apple, frozen seedless grapes, and kale leaves in a blender.
2. Cover and blend until it's smooth.
3. Smoothie is ready and can be garnished with halved grapes if you wish.

Nutrition:
- Calories: 81
- Protein: 2 g
- Carbohydrates: 19 g
- Fats: 1 g

224. Lean and Green Smoothie 2

Difficulty: Easy
Preparation Time: 5 minutes
Cooking Time: 0 minutes
Servings: 1
Ingredients:
- 6 kale leaves
- 2 peeled oranges
- 2 cups mango kombucha
- 2 cups chopped pineapple
- 2 cups water

Directions:
1. Break up the oranges, and place them in the blender.
2. Add the mango kombucha, chopped pineapple, and kale leaves into the blender.
3. Blend everything until it is smooth.
4. Smoothie is ready to be taken.

Nutrition:
- Calories: 81
- Protein: 2 g
- Carbohydrates: 19 g
- Fats: 1 g

225. Lean and Green Chicken Pesto Pasta

Difficulty: Easy
Preparation Time: 5 minutes
Cooking Time: 15 minutes
Servings: 1
Ingredients:
- 3 cups raw kale leaves
- 2 tbsp olive oil
- 2 cups fresh basil
- 1/4 tsp salt
- 3 tbsp lemon juice
- 3 garlic cloves
- 2 cups cooked chicken breast
- 1 cup baby spinach
- 6 ounces uncooked chicken pasta
- 3 ounces diced fresh mozzarella
- Basil leaves or red pepper flakes to garnish

Directions:
1. Start by making the pesto; add the kale, lemon juice, basil, garlic cloves, olive oil, and salt to a blender and blend until it's smooth.
2. Add salt and pepper to taste.
3. Cook the pasta and strain off the water. Reserve 1/4 cup of the liquid.
4. Get a bowl and mix everything, the cooked pasta, pesto, diced chicken, spinach, mozzarella, and the reserved pasta liquid.
5. Sprinkle the mixture with additional chopped basil or red paper flakes (optional).
6. Now your salad is ready. You may serve it warm or chilled. Also, it can be taken as a salad mix-in or as a side dish. Leftovers should be stored in the refrigerator inside an air-tight container for 3–5 days.

Nutrition:
- Calories: 244
- Protein: 20.5 g
- Carbohydrates: 22.5 g
- Fats: 10 g

226. Open-Face Egg Sandwiches with Cilantro-Jalapeño Spread

Difficulty: Intermediate
Preparation Time: 20 minutes
Cooking Time: 10 minutes
Servings: 2
Ingredients:
For the cilantro and jalapeño spread:
- 1 cup filled up fresh cilantro leaves and stems (about a bunch)
- 1 jalapeño pepper, seeded and roughly chopped
- ½ cup extra-virgin olive oil
- ¼ cup pepitas (hulled pumpkin seeds), raw or roasted
- 2 garlic cloves, thinly sliced
- 1 tbsp freshly squeezed lime juice
- 1 tsp kosher salt

For the eggs:
- 4 large eggs
- ¼ cup milk
- ¼ to ½ tsp kosher salt
- 2 tbsp butter

For the sandwich:
- 2 slices bread
- 1 tbsp butter
- 1 avocado, halved, pitted, and divided into slices
- Microgreens or sprouts, for garnish

Directions:
To make the cilantro and jalapeño spread:
1. In a food processor, combine the cilantro, jalapeño, oil, pepitas, garlic, lime juice, and salt. Whirl until smooth. Refrigerate if made in advance; otherwise set aside.

To make the eggs:
2. In a medium bowl, whisk the eggs, milk, and salt.
3. Dissolve the butter in a skillet over low heat, swirling to coat the bottom of the pan. Pour in the whisked eggs.
4. Cook until they begin to set then, using a heatproof spatula, push them to the sides, allowing the uncooked portions to run into the bottom of the skillet.
5. Continue until the eggs are set.

To assemble the sandwiches:
6. Toast the bed and spread with butter.
7. Spread a spoonful of the cilantro-jalapeño spread on each piece of toast. Top each with scrambled eggs.
8. Arrange avocado over each sandwich and garnish with microgreens.

Nutrition:
- Calories: 711
- Total fat: 4 g
- Cholesterol: 54 mg
- Fiber: 12 g
- Protein: 12 g
- Sodium: 327 mg

227. Alkaline Blueberry Spelt Pancakes

Difficulty: Easy
Preparation Time: 6 minutes
Cooking Time: 20 minutes
Servings: 3
Ingredients:
- 2 cups spelt flour
- 1 cup coconut milk
- 1/2 cup alkaline water
- 2 tbsp grapeseed oil
- 1/2 cup agave
- 1/2 cup blueberries
- 1/4 tsp sea moss

Directions:
1. Mix the spelt flour, agave, grapeseed oil, and sea moss in a bowl.
2. Add one cup of hemp milk and alkaline water to the mixture until you get the consistency you like.
3. Crimp the blueberries into the batter.
4. Heat the skillet to moderate heat then lightly coat it with the grapeseed oil.
5. Pour the batter into the skillet then let them cook for approximately 5 minutes on every side.
6. Serve and enjoy.

Nutrition:
- Calories: 203 kcal
- Fat: 1.4 g
- Carbs: 41.6 g
- Proteins: 4.8 g

228. Alkaline Blueberry Muffins

Difficulty: Easy
Preparation Time: 5 Minutes
Cooking Time: 20 minutes
Servings: 3
Ingredients:
- 1 cup coconut milk
- 3/4 cup spelt flour
- ¾ cup teff flour
- 1/2 cup blueberries
- 1/3 cup agave
- 1/4 cup sea moss gel
- 1/2 tsp sea salt
- Grapeseed oil

Directions:
1. Adjust the temperature of the oven to 365°F.
2. Grease six regular-size muffin cups with muffin liners.

3. In a bowl, mix sea salt, sea moss, agave, coconut milk, sea moss gel, and flour until they are properly blended.
4. You then crimp in blueberries.
5. Coat the muffin pan lightly with the grapeseed oil.
6. Pour in the muffin batter.
7. Bake for at least 30 minutes until they turn golden brown.
8. Serve.

Nutrition:
- Calories: 160 kcal
- Fat: 5 g
- Carbs: 25 g
- Proteins: 2 g

229. Crunchy Quinoa Meal

Difficulty: Easy
Preparation Time: 5 minutes
Cooking Time: 25 minutes
Servings: 2
Ingredients:
- 3 cups coconut milk
- 1 cup rinsed quinoa
- 1/8 tsp ground cinnamon
- 1 cup raspberry
- 1/2 cup chopped coconuts

Directions:
1. In a saucepan, pour the milk and bring it to a boil over moderate heat.
2. Add the quinoa to the milk and then bring it to a boil once more.
3. You then let it simmer for at least 15 minutes on medium heat until the milk is reduced.
4. Stir in the cinnamon, and then mix properly.
5. Cover it, and then cook for 8 minutes until the milk is completely absorbed.
6. Add the raspberry and cook the meal for 30 seconds.
7. Serve and enjoy.

Nutrition:
- Calories: 271 kcal
- Fat: 3.7 g
- Carbs: 54 g
- Proteins: 6.5 g

230. Coconut Pancakes

Difficulty: Easy
Preparation Time: 5 minutes
Cooking Time: 15 minutes
Servings: 4
Ingredients:
- 1 cup coconut flour
- 2 tbsp arrowroot powder
- 1 tsp baking powder
- 1 cup coconut milk
- 3 tbsp coconut oil

Directions:
1. In a medium container, mix in all the dry ingredients.
2. Add the coconut milk and two tbsp s. of the coconut oil then mix properly.
3. In a skillet, melt one tsp of coconut oil.
4. Pour a ladle of the batter into the skillet, then swirl the pan to spread the batter evenly into a smooth pancake.
5. Cook it for around three minutes on medium heat until it becomes firm.
6. Turn the pancake to the other side, then cook it for another 2 minutes until it turns golden brown.
7. Cook the remaining pancakes in the same process.
8. Serve.

Nutrition:
- Calories: 377 kcal
- Fat: 14.9 g
- Carbs: 60.7 g
- Protein: 6.4 g

231. Cashew Yogurt Bowl

Difficulty: Easy
Preparation Time: 5 minutes
Cooking Time: 0 minutes
Servings: 2
Ingredients:

- ¾ cup vegan cashew yogurt
- 1 tbsp flaxseed
- 1 tbsp chia seeds
- 1 tbsp hemp seed
- ¼ cup frozen blueberries

Directions:
1. Add the cashew yogurt to the bottom of the serving bowl.
2. Top with the remaining ingredients, going around steadily in a circle until all the ingredients are used up.
3. Serve.

Nutrition:
- Total Fat: 11.4 g
- Cholesterol: 0 mg
- Sodium: 18 mg
- Total Carbohydrates: 15.6 g
- Dietary fiber: 7.5 g
- Protein: 6.6 g
- Calcium: 180 mg
- Potassium: 170 mg
- Iron: 3 mg
- Vitamin D: 0 mcg

232. Zucchini Breakfast Bars

Difficulty: Medium
Preparation Time: 10 minutes
Cooking Time: 35 minutes
Servings: 6
Ingredients:

- 1 cup zucchini grated
- ¼ cup coconut butter, softened
- 2 tsp cinnamon
- 1 tbsp chia seeds
- ½ cup hemp hearts
- 2 tbsp granulated erythritol
- A pinch of salt

Directions:
1. Preheat your oven to 375°F.
2. Prepare a 9 x 13 loaf pan by lining it with parchment paper.
3. To a large mixing bowl, add coconut butter, zucchini, and erythritol. Combine thoroughly.
4. Add the rest of the ingredients and stir to thoroughly incorporate.
5. Allow the mixture to sit for 5 minutes so that the chia seeds thicken the batter.
6. Pour the mixture into a prepared pan and smooth the top with a spatula.
7. Bake for 35 minutes or until the bars are golden brown and firm to the touch.
8. Allow cooling for at least 30 minutes before removing from the. Slice into individual bars and serve.

Nutrition:
- Total Fat: 17 g
- Cholesterol: 0 mg
- Sodium: 35 mg
- Total Carbohydrates: 10 g
- Dietary fiber: 6.3 g
- Protein: 7.1 g
- Calcium: 56 mg
- Potassium: 77 mg
- Iron: 3 mg
- Vitamin D: 0 mcg

233. Cheesy Scrambled Tofu

Difficulty: Easy
Preparation Time: 10 minutes
Cooking Time: 15 minutes
Servings: 4
Ingredients:

- 14 oz. firm tofu
- 1 ½ tbsp nutritional yeast
- 3 oz. vegan cheddar cheese
- 1 medium tomato, diced
- 1 cup spinach
- ½ tsp salt
- ½ tsp turmeric
- ½ tsp garlic powder
- 3 tbsp olive oil

- 2 tbsp yellow onion, diced

Directions:
1. Wrap the block of tofu in a clean cloth towel and gently squeeze to remove excess moisture. Set aside.
2. Place a nonstick skillet over medium heat. Add 1/3 of the olive oil and add onions. Sauté until the onions become translucent.
3. Add the block of tofu to the skillet and crumble using a fork or potato masher. Do this until the tofu resembles scrambled eggs.
4. Add the remaining oil, nutritional yeast, garlic powder, turmeric and salt, and stir.
5. Cover the pot and continue to cook, stirring occasionally, until most of the moisture in the pot has evaporated.
6. Add spinach, tomato, and vegan cheese.
7. Cook for 1 more minute or until the spinach has wilted and the cheese is melted. Serve hot.
8. Can be stored in the refrigerator for up to three days in an airtight container.

Nutrition:
- Total Fat: 18.8 g
- Cholesterol: 0 mg
- Sodium: 418 mg
- Total Carbohydrates: 9.6 g
- Dietary fiber: 3.3 g
- Protein: 10.9 g
- Calcium: 215 mg
- Potassium: 373 mg
- Iron: 3 mg
- Vitamin D: 0 mcg

234. Zucchini Bacon Bake

Difficulty: Easy
Preparation Time: 10 minutes
Cooking Time: 30 minutes
Servings: 8
Ingredients:
- 8 egg whites
- 3 tbsp bacon, crumbled
- 1/4 cup unsweetened almond milk
- 3 wedges Swiss cheese
- 1/2 cup cottage cheese
- 2 cups shredded zucchini
- 1/2 tsp salt

Directions:
1. Preheat the oven to 350°F.
2. Grease 8*8-inch casserole dish.
3. Add shredded zucchini into the prepared dish.
4. Add egg, bacon, milk, Swiss cheese, cottage cheese, and salt into the blender and blend until smooth.
5. Pour the blended egg mixture over shredded zucchini.
6. Bake in preheated oven for 30 minutes.
7. Serve and enjoy.

Nutrition:
- Calories: 114
- Fat: 6.4 g
- Carbohydrates: 2.4 g
- Sugar 0.9 g
- Protein 11.4 g
- Cholesterol 19 mg

235. Cauliflower Breakfast Casserole

Difficulty: Intermediate
Preparation Time: 10 minutes
Cooking Time: 45 minutes
Servings: 6
Ingredients:
- 10 eggs
- 4 cups cauliflower rice
- 12 oz. bacon, cooked and crumbled
- 1/2 cup heavy whipping cream
- 1 tsp paprika
- 8 oz. cheddar cheese, shredded
- 1/4 tsp pepper
- 1 tsp salt

Directions:
1. Preheat the oven to 350°F.
2. Grease 2-quart casserole dish.
3. Spread cauliflower rice into the prepared dish and top with half cheddar cheese.
4. In a bowl, whisk eggs with cream, paprika, pepper, and salt and pour over cauliflower.
5. Top with the remaining cheese and bacon.

6. Bake for 45 minutes.
7. Serve and enjoy.

Nutrition:
- Calories: 637
- Fat: 48.5 g
- Carbohydrates: 6.9 g
- Sugar 3.5 g
- Protein 42.5 g
- Cholesterol 389 mg

236. Jalapeno Breakfast Casserole

Difficulty: Easy
Preparation Time: 10 minutes
Cooking Time: 30 minutes
Servings: 10
Ingredients:
- 12 eggs
- 2 jalapeno peppers, sliced
- 4 oz. cream cheese, cut into cubes
- 1 cup cheddar cheese, shredded
- 1/2 cup bacon, cooked and chopped
- 1 cup heavy whipping cream
- 1/2 tsp pepper
- 1/4 tsp salt

Directions:
1. Preheat the oven to 350°F. Grease a 9x13-inch baking pan and set it aside.
2. In a large bowl, whisk eggs with cream cheese, cream, pepper, and salt and pour into the prepared pan.
3. Sprinkle jalapeno slices, bacon, and 3/4 cup cheddar cheese evenly over the egg mixture.
4. Bake for 25–30 minutes. Remove pan from oven and top with the remaining cheese and bake for 5 minutes more.
5. Serve and enjoy.

Nutrition:
- Calories: 209
- Fat: 17.8 g
- Carbohydrates: 1.5 g
- Sugar: 0.6 g
- Protein: 11 g
- Cholesterol 238 mg

237. Easy Cheese Egg Bake

Difficulty: Easy
Preparation Time: 10 minutes
Cooking Time: 30 minutes
Servings: 4
Ingredients:
- 4 eggs
- 1/3 cup half and half
- 4 oz. cream cheese
- A pinch of salt

Directions:
1. Preheat the oven to 350°F.
2. Add eggs, half and half, cream cheese, and salt into the blender and blend until smooth.
3. Pour the egg mixture into the greased baking dish and bake for 30 minutes.
4. Serve and enjoy.

Nutrition:
- Calories: 188
- Fat: 16.6 g
- Carbohydrates: 2 g
- Sugar: 0.4 g
- Protein: 8.3 g
- Cholesterol: 202 mg

238. Sausage Egg Omelet

Difficulty: Easy
Preparation Time: 10 minutes
Cooking Time: 23 minutes
Servings: 12
Ingredients:
- 7 eggs
- 1 tsp mustard
- 2 cups cheddar cheese, shredded
- 3/4 cup heavy whipping cream
- 1/4 onion, chopped
- 1/2 green bell pepper, chopped
- 1 lb. breakfast sausage
- 1/4 tsp pepper
- 1/2 tsp salt

Directions:
1. Preheat the oven to 350°F. Grease 9*13-inch casserole dish and set aside.

2. Brown the sausage in a pan. Add onion and bell pepper and cook until the onion is softened. Remove pan from heat.
3. In a bowl, whisk eggs with mustard, 1 3/4 cups of cheese, cream, pepper, and salt.
4. Spread the sausage mixture into the prepared casserole. Pour the egg mixture on top of the sausage mixture and top with the remaining cheese.
5. Bake for 20–23 minutes.
6. Serve and enjoy.

Nutrition:
- Calories: 271
- Fat: 22.4 g
- Carbohydrates: 1.4 g
- Sugar: 0.7 g
- Protein: 15.6 g
- Cholesterol: 157 mg

239. Broccoli Egg Bake

Difficulty: Medium
Preparation Time: 10 minutes
Cooking Time: 30 minutes
Servings: 6
Ingredients:
- 12 eggs
- 2 cups broccoli florets, chopped
- 1/2 cup cheddar cheese, shredded
- 3/4 tsp onion powder
- 1/2 cup unsweetened coconut milk
- Pepper
- Salt

Directions:
1. Preheat the oven to 350°F. Grease 9*13-inch baking dish.
2. In a bowl, whisk eggs with cheese, onion powder, milk, pepper, and salt. Stir in broccoli.
3. Pour the egg mixture into the prepared dish and bake for 30 minutes.
4. Slice and serve.

Nutrition:
- Calories: 221
- Fat: 16.7 g
- Carbohydrates: 4.2 g
- Sugar: 2 g
- Protein: 14.8 g
- Cholesterol: 337 mg

240. Chicken Cheese Quiche

Difficulty: Medium
Preparation Time: 10 minutes
Cooking Time: 45 minutes
Servings: 4
Ingredients:
- 8 eggs
- 1/2 tsp oregano
- 1/4 tsp onion powder
- 1/4 tsp garlic powder
- 1/4 cup mozzarella cheese, shredded
- 5 oz. cooked chicken breast, chopped
- 1/4 tsp pepper
- 1/2 tsp salt

Directions:
1. Preheat the oven to 350°F.
2. In a bowl, whisk eggs with oregano, onion powder, pepper, and salt. Stir in cheese and chicken.
3. Pour the egg mixture into a pie pan and bake for 35–45 minutes.
4. Slice and serve.

Nutrition:
- Calories: 173
- Fat: 10 g
- Carbohydrates: 1.2 g
- Sugar: 0.8 g
- Protein: 19.2 g
- Cholesterol: 351 mg

241. Egg & Bacon Cups

Difficulty: Easy
Preparation Time: 10 minutes
Cooking Time: 15 minutes
Servings: 6
Ingredients:
- 2 bacon strips
- 2 large eggs
- A handful fresh spinach
- ¼ cup cheese

- Salt and pepper to taste

Directions:
1. Preheat your oven to 400°F.
2. Fry the bacon in a skillet over medium heat, drain the oil and keep them on the side.
3. Take muffin tin and grease with oil.
4. Line with a slice of bacon and press down the bacon well, making sure that the ends are sticking out (to be used as handles).
5. Take a bowl and beat eggs.
6. Drain and pat the spinach dry.
7. Add the spinach to the eggs.
8. Add a quarter of the mixture to each of your muffin tins.
9. Sprinkle cheese and season.
10. Bake for 15 minutes.
11. Enjoy!

Nutrition:
- Calories: 101
- Fat: 7 g
- Carbohydrates: 2 g
- Protein: 8 g
- Fiber: 1 g
- Net Carbs: 1 g

242. **Cottage Cheese Hotcake**

Difficulty: Easy
Preparation Time: 10 minutes
Cooking Time: 5–10 minutes
Servings: 2
Ingredients:
- 1 cup full-fat cottage cheese
- ½ cup full-fat ricotta cheese
- 2 whole eggs
- ¼ cup coconut cream
- ½ tsp baking powder
- 1 tsp vanilla extract
- Butter for frying
- 2 tsp almond butter

Directions:
1. Add cottage cheese, ricotta cheese, eggs, and coconut cream to a bowl. Whisk well.
2. Add ground almond, coconut flour, baking powder, vanilla extra, and whisk until smooth.
3. Preheat the non-stick frying pan over medium heat.
4. Add a knob of butter.
5. Once butter melts, add dollops of batter onto a hot pan.
6. Once bubbles appear, flip the pancakes over.
7. Serve with almond butter.
8. Enjoy!

Nutrition:
- Calories: 690
- Fat: 48 g
- Carbohydrates: 16 g
- Protein: 40 g
- Fiber: 3 g
- Net Carbohydrates: 13 g

243. **Chard Omelet**

Difficulty: Easy
Preparation Time: 5 minutes
Cooking Time: 5 minutes
Servings: 2
Ingredients:
- 2 eggs, lightly beaten
- 2 cups Swiss chard, sliced
- 1 tbsp butter
- ½ tsp garlic salt
- Fresh pepper

Directions:
1. Take a non-stick frying pan and place it over medium-low heat.
2. Once the butter melts, add Swiss chard and stir cook for 2 minutes.
3. Pour egg into the pan and gently stir them into Swiss chard.
4. Season with garlic salt and pepper.
5. Cook for 2 minutes.
6. Serve and enjoy!

Nutrition:
- Calories: 260
- Fat: 21 g
- Net Carbohydrates: 4 g
- Protein: 14 g
- Fiber: 1 g
- Carbohydrates: 5 g

244. Scrambled Pesto Eggs

Difficulty: Easy
Preparation Time: 5 minutes
Cooking Time: 5 minutes
Servings: 2
Ingredients:
- 2 large whole eggs
- 1/2 tbsp butter
- 1/2 tbsp pesto
- 1 tbsp creamed coconut milk
- Salt, as needed
- Pepper, as needed

Directions:
1. Take a bowl and crack open your egg.
2. Sprinkle with salt and pepper to your taste.
3. Pour eggs into a pan.
4. Add butter and introduce heat.
5. Cook on low heat and gently add pesto.
6. Once the egg is cooked and scrambled, remove it from the heat.
7. Spoon in coconut cream and mix well.
8. Turn on the heat and cook on LOW for a while until you have a creamy texture.
9. Serve and enjoy!

Nutrition:
- Calories: 467
- Fat: 41 g
- Carbohydrates: 3 g
- Protein: 20 g
- Fiber: 2 g
- Net Carbohydrates: 1 g

245. Devil Eggs

Difficulty: Easy
Preparation Time: 9 minutes
Cooking Time: 11 minutes
Servings: 2
Ingredients:
- 4 whole hard-boiled eggs
- 2 tbsp mayonnaise (Keto friendly or homemade)
- 1 tbsp spicy brown mustard
- 1 tbsp green chilies, diced

Directions:
1. Boil your eggs for 9 minutes.
2. Transfer boiled eggs to a water bath and peel the skin.
3. Slice the egg in half and scoop out the yolks.
4. Take a bowl and add yolks, mayonnaise, chilies, and mustard.
5. Mix well and transfer the mixture back to the egg white shells.
6. Enjoy!

Nutrition:
- Calories: 202
- Fat: 15 g
- Net Carbohydrates: 3 g
- Protein: 12 g
- Fiber: 2 g
- Carbohydrates: 5 g

246. Asparagus & Crabmeat Frittata

Difficulty: Easy
Preparation Time: 5 minutes
Cooking Time: 15 minutes
Servings: 4
Ingredients:
- 2½ tbsp extra virgin olive oil
- 2 lb. asparagus
- 1 tsp salt
- 1 ½ tsp black pepper
- 2 tsp sweet paprika
- 1 lb. lump crabmeat
- 1 tbsp finely cut chives
- ¼ cup basil chopped
- 4 cups liquid egg substitute

Directions:
1. Deter the tough ends of the asparagus and cut it into bite-sized pieces.
2. Preheat an oven to 375°F.
3. In a 12-Inch to a 14-inch oven-proof, non-stick skillet, warm the olive oil and sweat the asparagus until tender. Season with pepper, paprika, and salt.
4. In a mixing bowl, add the chives, crab, and basil meat.

5. Pour in the liquid egg substitute and mix until combined.
6. Pour the crab and egg mixture into the skillet with the cooked asparagus and stir to combine.
7. Bake over low to medium heat until the eggs start bubbling.
8. Place the skillet in the oven and bake for about 15–20 minutes until the eggs are golden brown. Serve the dish warm.

Nutrition:
- Calories: 340
- Protein: 50 g
- Carbohydrate: 14 g
- Fat: 10 g

247. Bacon Cheeseburger

Difficulty: Easy
Preparation Time: 5 minutes
Cooking Time: 15 minutes
Servings: 4
Ingredients:
- 1 lb. lean ground beef
- ¼ cup chopped yellow onion
- 1 garlic clove, minced
- 1 tbsp yellow mustard
- 1 tbsp Worcestershire sauce
- ½ tsp salt
- Cooking spray
- 4 ultra-thin slices cheddar cheese, cut into 6 equal-sized rectangular pieces
- 3 pieces of turkey bacon, each cut into 8 evenly-sized rectangular pieces
- 24 dill pickle chips
- 4–6 green leaf lettuce leaves, torn into 24 small square-shaped pieces
- 12 cherry tomatoes, sliced in half

Directions:
1. Pre-heat oven to 400°F.
2. Combine the garlic, salt, onion, Worcestershire sauce, and beef in a medium-sized bowl, and mix well.
3. Form the mixture into 24 small meatballs. Put meatballs onto a foil-lined baking sheet and cook for 12–15 minutes. Leave oven on.
4. Top every meatball with a piece of cheese, then go back to the oven till the cheese melts, about 2 to 3 minutes. Let meatballs cool.
5. To assemble bites: on a toothpick layer a cheese-covered meatball, piece of bacon, piece of lettuce, pickle chip, and a tomato half.

Nutrition:
- Calories: 234
- Protein: 20 g
- Fat: 3 g
- Carbs: 12 g

248. Ancho Tilapia on Cauliflower Rice

Difficulty: Intermediate
Preparation Time: 15 minutes
Cooking Time: 30 minutes
Servings: 4
Ingredients:
- 2 lb. tilapia
- 1 tsp lime juice
- 1 tsp salt
- 1 tbsp ground ancho pepper
- 1 tsp ground cumin
- 1 ½ tbsp extra virgin olive oil
- ¼ cup toasted pumpkin seeds
- 6 cups cauliflower rice minutes
- 1 cup coarsely chopped fresh cilantro

Directions:
1. Preheat the oven to 450°F.
2. Dress tilapia with lime juice and set aside.
3. Combine cumin, ancho pepper, and salt in a bowl. Season tilapia with spice mixture.
4. Lay tilapia on a baking sheet or casserole dish and bake for 7 minutes.
5. In the meantime, in a big skillet, sweat the cauliflower rice in olive oil till tender, about 2–3 minutes.
6. Blend the pumpkin seeds and cilantro into the rice. Dismiss from heat, and serve.

Nutrition:
- Calories: 350
- Fat: 13 g
- Carbohydrate: 10 g

- Protein: 51 g

249. Turkey Caprese Meatloaf Cups

Difficulty: Medium
Preparation Time: 20 minutes
Cooking Time: 45 minutes
Servings: 6
Ingredients:
- 1 large egg
- 2 pounds ground turkey breast
- 3 pieces of sun-dried tomatoes, drained and chopped
- ¼ cup fresh basil leaves, chopped
- 5 ounces low-fat fresh mozzarella, shredded
- ½ tsp garlic powder
- ¼ tsp salt and
- ½ tsp pepper, to taste

Directions:
1. Preheat the oven to 400°F.
2. Beat the egg in a big mixing bowl.
3. Add the remaining ingredients and mix everything with your hands until evenly combined.
4. Spray a 12-cup muffin tin and divide the turkey mixture among the muffin cups, pressing the mix in.
5. Cook in the preheated oven till the turkey is well-cooked for about 25–30 minutes.
6. Chill the meatloaves entirely and store them in a container in the fridge for up to 5 days.

Nutrition:
- Calories: 181
- Protein 43 g
- Fat: 11 g
- Carbs: 9 g

250. Cinnamon Coconut Porridge

Difficulty: Easy
Preparation Time: 5 minutes
Cooking Time: 0 minutes
Servings: 1
Ingredients:
- 2 tbsp shredded coconut
- 1 tbsp ground flax seeds
- 2 tbsp hemp hearts
- ⅛ tsp cinnamon
- ⅛ tsp stevia powder
- ½ cup boiling water
- Fresh mixed berries to top

Directions:
1. Add all the ingredients except for fresh mixed berries and water to a serving bowl and stir to combine.
2. Add boiling water. Stir.
3. Allow the porridge to sit until it reaches a suitable eating temperature.
4. The porridge will thicken as it cools down.
5. Top with fresh mixed berries and serve.

Nutrition:
- Total Fat: 31.5 g
- Cholesterol: 0 mg
- Sodium: 8 mg
- Total Carbohydrates: 9.8 g
- Dietary fiber: 9 g
- Protein: 21.7 g
- Calcium: 49 mg
- Potassium: 95 mg
- Iron: 11 mg
- Vitamin D: 0 mcg

LUNCH RECIPES

251. Bacon-Wrapped Asparagus

Difficulty: Intermediate
Preparation Time: 10 minutes
Cooking Time: 20 minutes
Servings: 2
Ingredients:

- 1/3 cup heavy whipping cream
- 2 bacon slices, precooked
- 4 small spears asparagus
- Salt, to taste
- 1 tbsp butter

Directions:

1. Preheat the oven to 360°F and grease a baking sheet with butter.
2. Meanwhile, mix cream, asparagus, and salt in a bowl.
3. Wrap the asparagus in bacon slices and arrange them in the baking dish.
4. Transfer the baking dish to the oven and bake for about 20 minutes.
5. Remove from the oven and serve hot.
6. Place the bacon-wrapped asparagus in a dish and set it aside to cool for meal prepping. Divide it into 2 containers and cover the lid. Refrigerate for about 2 days and reheat in the microwave before serving.

Nutrition:

- Calories: 204
- Carbs: 1.4 g
- Protein: 5.9 g
- Fat: 19.3 g
- Sugar: 0.5 g

252. Spinach Chicken

Difficulty: Easy
Preparation Time: 10 minutes
Cooking Time: 10 minutes
Servings: 2
Ingredients:

- 2 garlic cloves, minced
- 2 tbsp unsalted butter, divided
- ¼ cup parmesan cheese, shredded
- ¾ pound chicken tenders
- ¼ cup heavy cream
- 10 ounces frozen spinach, chopped
- Salt and black pepper, to taste

Directions:

1. Heat 1 tbsp of butter in a large skillet and add chicken, salt, and black pepper.
2. Cook for about 3 minutes on both sides and remove the chicken to a bowl.
3. Melt the remaining butter in the skillet and add garlic, cheese, heavy cream, and spinach.
4. Cook for about 2 minutes and add the chicken.
5. Cook for about 5 minutes on low heat and dish out to immediately serve.
6. Place chicken in a dish and set aside to cool for meal prepping. Divide it into 2 containers and cover them. Refrigerate for about 3 days and reheat in the microwave before serving.

Nutrition:

- Calories: 288
- Carbs: 3.6 g
- Protein: 27.7 g
- Fat: 18.3 g
- Sugar: 0.3 g

253. Lemongrass Prawns

Difficulty: Easy
Preparation Time: 10 minutes
Cooking Time: 15 minutes
Servings: 2
Ingredients:

- ½ red chili pepper, seeded and chopped
- 2 lemongrass stalks
- ½ pound prawns, deveined and peeled
- 6 tbsp butter
- ¼ tsp smoked paprika

Directions:

1. Preheat the oven to 390°F and grease a baking dish.

2. Mix red chili pepper, butter, smoked paprika, and prawns in a bowl.
3. Marinate for about 2 hours and then thread the prawns on the lemongrass stalks.
4. Arrange the threaded prawns on the baking dish and transfer them to the oven.
5. Bake for about 15 minutes and dish out to serve immediately.
6. Place the prawns in a dish and set them aside to cool for meal prepping. Divide it into 2 containers and close the lid. Refrigerate for about 4 days and reheat in the microwave before serving.

Nutrition:
- Calories: 322
- Carbs: 3.8 g
- Protein: 34.8 g
- Fat: 18 g
- Sugar: 0.1 g
- Sodium: 478 mg

254. **Stuffed Mushrooms**

Difficulty: Easy
Preparation Time: 20 minutes
Cooking Time: 25 minutes
Servings: 2
Ingredients:
- 2 ounces bacon, crumbled
- ½ tbsp butter
- ¼ tsp paprika powder
- 2 Portobello mushrooms
- 1 oz. cream cheese
- ¾ tbsp fresh chives, chopped
- Salt and black pepper, to taste

Directions:
1. Preheat the oven to 400°F and grease a baking dish.
2. Heat butter in a skillet and add mushrooms.
3. Sauté for about 4 minutes and set aside.
4. Mix cream cheese, chives, paprika powder, salt, and black pepper in a bowl.
5. Stuff the mushrooms with this mixture and transfer them to the baking dish.
6. Place in the oven and bake for about 20 minutes.
7. These mushrooms can be refrigerated for about 3 days for meal prepping and can be served with scrambled eggs.

Nutrition:
- Calories: 570
- Carbs: 4.6 g
- Protein: 19.9 g
- Fat: 52.8 g
- Sugar: 0.8 g
- Sodium: 1041 mg

255. **Keto Zucchini Pizza**

Difficulty: Easy
Preparation Time: 10 minutes
Cooking Time: 15 minutes
Servings: 2
Ingredients:
- 1/8 cup spaghetti sauce
- ½ zucchini, cut into circular slices
- ½ cup cream cheese
- Pepperoni slices, for topping
- ½ cup mozzarella cheese, shredded

Directions:
1. Preheat the oven to 350°F and grease a baking dish.
2. Arrange the zucchini on the baking dish and layer with spaghetti sauce.
3. Top with pepperoni slices and mozzarella cheese.
4. Transfer the baking dish to the oven and bake for about 15 minutes.
5. Remove from the oven and serve immediately.

Nutrition:
- Calories: 445
- Carbs: 3.6 g
- Protein: 12.8 g
- Fat: 42 g
- Sugar: 0.3 g
- Sodium: 429 mg

256. Crab Cakes

Difficulty: Easy
Preparation Time: 20 minutes
Cooking Time: 10 minutes
Servings: 2
Ingredients:

- ½ pound lump crabmeat, drained
- 2 tbsp coconut flour
- 1 tbsp mayonnaise
- ¼ tsp green Tabasco sauce
- 3 tbsp butter
- 1 small egg, beaten
- ¾ tbsp fresh parsley, chopped
- ½ tsp yellow mustard
- Salt and black pepper, to taste

Directions:
1. Mix all the ingredients in a bowl except butter.
2. Make patties from this mixture and set them aside.
3. Heat butter in a skillet over medium heat and add patties.
4. Cook for about 10 minutes on each side and dish out to serve hot.
5. You can store the raw patties in the freezer for about 3 weeks for meal prepping. Place patties in a container and place parchment paper in between the patties to avoid stickiness.

Nutrition:

- Calories: 153
- Fat: 10.8 g
- Carbs: 6.7 g
- Protein: 6.4 g
- Sugar: 2.4 g
- Sodium: 46 mg

257. Low Carb Black Beans Chili Chicken

Difficulty: Easy
Preparation Time: 10 minutes
Cooking Time: 25 minutes
Servings: 10
Ingredients:

- 1-3/4 pounds chicken breasts, cubed (boneless skinless)
- 2 sweet red peppers, chopped
- 1 onion, chopped
- 3 tbsp olive oil
- 1 can chopped green chiles
- 4 garlic cloves, minced
- 2 tbsp chili powder
- 2 tsp ground cumin
- 1 tsp ground coriander
- 2 cans black beans, rinsed and drained
- 1 can Italian stewed tomatoes, cut up
- 1 cup chicken broth or beer
- 1/2 to 1 cup water

Directions:
1. Put oil into a skillet and place over medium heat. Add in the red pepper, chicken, and onion, and cook until the chicken is brown for about five minutes.
2. Add in the garlic, chiles, chili powder, coriander, and cumin, and cook for an additional minute.
3. Next, add in the tomatoes, beans, half cup of water, and broth, and cook until it boils. Decrease the heat, uncover the skillet and cook while stirring for fifteen minutes.
4. Serve.

Nutrition:

- Calories: 236
- Fat: 6 g
- Protein: 22 g
- Carbohydrates: 21 g

258. Quick Keto BLT Chicken Salad

Difficulty: Easy
Preparation Time: 20 minutes
Cooking Time: 0 minutes
Servings: 8
Ingredients:

- 1/2 cup mayonnaise
- 3 to 4 tbsp barbecue sauce
- 2 tbsp finely chopped onion
- 1 tbsp lemon juice

- 1/4 tsp pepper
- 8 cups torn salad greens
- 2 tomatoes, chopped
- 10 strips bacon, cooked and crumbled
- 2 hard-boiled eggs, sliced
- 1 1/2 pounds boneless skinless chicken breasts, cooked and cubed

Directions:
1. Mix the first five ingredients in a bowl until combined.
2. Cover the bowl and transfer the mixture to the refrigerator.
3. Next, put the salad greens in a bowl. Add in the chicken, tomatoes, and bacon.
4. Top with eggs and a drizzle of the dressing.
5. Serve.

Nutrition:
- Calories: 281
- Protein: 23 g
- Fat: 19 g
- Carbohydrates: 5 g

259. Quick Healthy Avocado Tuna Salad

Difficulty: Medium
Preparation Time: 10 minutes
Cooking Time: 0 minutes
Servings: 4
Ingredients:
- 2 Avocados
- 2 tbsp Lime juice
- 4 5-oz. cans Tuna, drained
- 1/4 cup fresh cilantro, chopped
- 3 tbsp celery, finely chopped
- 3 tbsp Red onion, minced
- 1 tbsp Jalapenos, minced
- 1/2 tsp Sea salt

Directions:
1. Crush the lime juice and avocado in a bowl. Add in the sea salt and combine.
2. Next, add in the cilantro, tuna, celery, red onion, and jalapenos.
3. Stir to combine. Adjust seasonings as desired and serve.

Nutrition:
- Calories: 169
- Protein: 27 g
- Fat: 14 g
- Carbohydrates: 10 g

260. Flavorful Keto Taco Soup

Difficulty: Easy
Preparation Time: 5 minutes
Cooking Time: 15
Servings: 8
Ingredients:
- 1 lb. Ground beef
- 3 tbsp taco seasoning, divided
- 4 cup Beef bone broth
- 2 14.5-oz. cans diced tomatoes
- 3/4 cup Ranch dressing

Directions:
1. Put the ground beef into a pot and place over medium-high heat and cook until brown, about ten minutes.
2. Add in ¾ cup of broth and two tbsp of taco seasoning. Cook until part of the liquid has evaporated.
3. Add in the diced tomatoes, rest of the broth, and rest of the taco seasoning. Stir to mix, then simmer for ten minutes.
4. Remove the pot from heat, and add the ranch dressing. Garnish with cilantro and cheddar cheese. Serve.

Nutrition:
- Calories: 309
- Fat: 24 g
- Protein: 13 g

261. Delicious Instant Pot Keto Buffalo Chicken Soup

Difficulty: Intermediate
Preparation Time: 10 minutes
Cooking Time: 20 minutes
Servings: 6
Ingredients:
- 1 tbsp Olive oil
- 1/2 Onion, diced
- 1/2 cup Celery, diced
- 4 Garlic cloves, minced
- 1 lb. Shredded chicken, cooked
- 4 cup chicken bone broth, or any chicken broth
- 3 tbsp buffalo sauce
- 6 oz. Cream cheese
- 1/2 cup half & half

Directions:
1. Switch the instant pot to the sauté function. Add in the chopped onion, oil, and celery. Cook until the onions are brown and translucent, about ten minutes.
2. Add in the garlic and cook until fragrant, about one minute. Switch off the instant pot.
3. Add in the broth, shredded chicken, and buffalo sauce. Cover the instant pot and seal. Switch the soup feature on and set the time to five minutes.
4. When cooked, release pressure naturally for five minutes and then quickly.
5. Scoop out one cup of the soup liquid into a blender bowl, then add in the cheese and blend until smooth. Pour the puree into the instant pot, then add in the calf and half and stir to mix.
6. Serve.

Nutrition:
- Calories: 270
- Protein: 27 g
- Fat: 16 g
- Carbohydrates: 4 g

262. Creamy Low Carb Cream of Mushroom Soup

Difficulty: Easy
Preparation Time: 15 minutes
Cooking Time: 15 minutes
Servings: 5
Ingredients:
- 1 tbsp Olive oil
- 1/2 Onion, diced
- 20 oz. Mushrooms, sliced
- 6 Garlic cloves, minced
- 2 cups Chicken broth
- 1 cup Heavy cream
- 1 cup unsweetened almond milk
- 3/4 tsp Sea salt
- 1/4 tsp Black pepper

Directions:
1. Place a pot over medium heat and add olive oil. Add the mushrooms and onions and cook until browned, about fifteen minutes. Next, add the garlic and cook for another one minute.
2. Add in the cream, chicken broth, sea salt, almond milk, and black pepper. Cook until boil, then simmer for fifteen minutes.
3. Puree the soup using an immersion blender until smooth. Serve.

Nutrition:
- Calories: 229
- Fat: 21 g
- Protein: 5 g
- Carbohydrates: 8 g

263. Easy Keto Chicken Soup

Difficulty: Easy
Preparation Time: 10 minutes
Cooking Time: 1 hour
Servings: 14
Ingredients:
- 2 cups shredded chicken, cooked
- 1 cup Carrots, diced
- 1 cup Celery, diced
- 1 cup Onion, diced
- 10 cups Chicken broth

- 1 tbsp Italian seasoning
- 1 Bay leaf
- A dash Sea salt
- A dash Black pepper
- 1 Spaghetti squash

Directions:
1. Combine all the ingredients minus the spaghetti squash in a pot over medium heat. Cook until it boils, then decrease to a simmer and cover the pot. Cook for one hour.
2. Next, preheat the oven to about 375°F, then punch holes in the spaghetti squash with a knife. Transfer to a baking sheet and bake in the oven for sixty minutes.
3. When the spaghetti squash is cooked, cut it in half and scoop out the strands using a fork. Remove the bay leaf and add in half of the spaghetti squash strands.

Nutrition:
- Calories: 44
- Carbohydrates: 4 g
- Protein: 5 g
- Fat: 1 g

264. Taco Casserole

Difficulty: Easy
Preparation Time: 30 minutes
Cooking Time: 1 Hour
Servings: 8
Ingredients:
- 1 lb. Ground Turkey
- 1 Cauliflower, Small & Chopped into Florets
- 1 Jalapeno Diced
- ¼ Cup Red Peppers, Diced
- ¼ Cup Onion, Diced
- 1 tsp Cumin
- 1 tsp Parsley
- 1 tsp Garlic Minced
- 1 tsp Turmeric
- 1 tsp Oregano
- 1 ½ Cups Cheddar Cheese, Shredded
- 1 cup Sour Cream

Directions:
1. Put your minced meat and cauliflower in a bowl before adding all your herbs and spices. Stir in your red peppers, jalapenos, and onions together, mixing in a cup of your cheese.
2. Pour into a casserole dish before topping with the remaining cheese.
3. Bake at 350°F for 1 hour and serve with sour cream.

Nutrition:
- Calories: 242
- Protein: 18 g
- Fat: 17 g
- Net Carbs: 4 g

265. Quick Keto Roasted Tomato Soup

Difficulty: Medium
Preparation Time: 5 minutes
Cooking Time: 40 minutes
Servings: 6
Ingredients:
- 10 fresh Rome tomatoes, sliced into tubes
- 2 tbsp Olive oil
- 4 Garlic cloves, minced
- 2 cups Chicken bone broth
- 1 tbsp Herbs de Provence
- 1/2 tsp Sea salt
- 1/4 tsp Black pepper
- 1/4 cup Heavy cream
- 2 tbsp fresh basil

Directions:
1. First, preheat the oven to about 400°F, then line a baking sheet with some foil, then grease the foil.
2. Mix the tomato chunks with minced garlic and olive oil. Place the tomato chunks on a baking sheet.
3. Transfer to the oven and bake until the skin wrinkles, about twenty-five minutes.
4. Remove from the heat and put the tomato chunks into the blender and blend until smooth.
5. Pour the tomato puree into the pot and place over medium-high heat. Add in the broth and season with sea salt, herbs de Provence, and black pepper. Boil for about fifteen minutes.

6. Add in the basil and cream and serve.

Nutrition:
- Calories: 95
- Fat: 8 g
- Protein: 3 g
- Carbohydrates: 3 g

266. **Delicious Low Carb Chicken Caesar Salad**

Difficulty: Intermediate
Preparation Time: 10 minutes
Cooking Time: 6 minutes
Servings: 4
Ingredients:
- 1 cup Parmesan crisps
- 1 head Romaine lettuce, chopped
- 2 cups Grape tomatoes, halved
- 2 grilled chicken breasts, sliced

For Keto Caesar Dressing:
- 1/3 cup Caesar salad dressing

Directions:
1. Chill the Caesar salad dressing in the refrigerator.
2. Combine the grape tomatoes, romaine lettuce, and cooked chicken.
3. Break the cheese crisps into bits and sprinkle on the salad and drizzle with the dressing. Mix to combine.

Nutrition:
- Calories: 400
- Protein: 33 g
- Fat: 25 g
- Carbohydrates: 5 g

267. **Keto Cheesy Broccoli Soup**

Difficulty: Easy
Preparation Time: 15 minutes
Cooking Time: 20 minutes
Servings: 8
Ingredients:
- 4 cups Broccoli, chopped into florets
- 4 Garlic cloves, minced
- 3 1/2 cups Chicken broth
- 1 cup Heavy cream
- 3 cups Cheddar cheese

Directions:
1. Place a pot over medium heat, then add in the garlic and cook until fragrant. Add in the heavy cream, chicken broth, and chopped broccoli.
2. Raise the heat and cook until it boils, then decrease the heat. Cook until the broccoli is tender, about twenty minutes.
3. Remove one-third of the broccoli and keep it aside. Blend the rest of the broccoli using an immersion blender. Decrease the heat to low.
4. Add in the cheddar cheese and stir until combined. Blend again to smooth.
5. Remove from the heat source, then add in the reserved broccoli florets and serve.

Nutrition:
- Calories: 292
- Protein: 13 g
- Fat: 25 g
- Carbohydrates: 5 g

268. **Creamy Low Carb Zucchini Alfredo**

Difficulty: Intermediate
Preparation Time: 10 minutes
Cooking Time: 15 minutes
Servings: 4
Ingredients:
- 3 Zucchini
- 1 tsp Butter
- 2 Garlic cloves, minced
- 1/4 tsp Nutmeg
- 1/2 cup unsweetened almond milk
- 1/3 cup Heavy cream
- 3/4 cup grated Parmesan cheese
- 1 tbsp Arrowroot powder
- A dash Black pepper

Directions:
1. First, prepare the zucchini noodles using a julienne peeler or spiralizer. Next, put butter into a skillet and place over medium-high heat. When heated, add in the garlic and cook until fragrant and soft, about a minute.

2. Decrease the heat to low heat, then add in the heavy cream, almond milk, and nutmeg. Boil for some minutes.
3. Combine the arrowroot powder with two tbsp of water in a bowl until dissolved, then pour into the sauce in the skillet.
4. Add in the Parmesan cheese and season with black pepper. Keep cooking while stirring frequently until the cheese melts. Transfer the sauce to a container and keep it aside.
5. Dry the zucchini using paper towels, then put the noodles into the pan and stir fry over medium-high heat. Cook until softened, about four minutes.
6. Pour in the sauce and garnish with more Parmesan cheese and parsley. Serve.

Nutrition:
- Calories: 209
- Protein: 11 g
- Fat: 16 g
- Carbohydrates: 9 g

269. <u>Amazing Low Carb Shrimp Lettuce Wraps.</u>

Difficulty: Easy
Preparation Time: 10 minutes
Cooking Time: 4 minutes
Servings: 4
Ingredients:
For Thai Shrimp:
- 1 lb. Shrimp, peeled, deveined
- 2 tbsp Coconut aminos
- 1/4 cup Olive oil, divided
- 1 tbsp Fish sauce
- 2 tsp Lime juice
- 1/4 tsp crushed red pepper flakes

For Lettuce Wraps:
- 16 leaves Bibb lettuce
- 1/3 fresh Cucumber, julienned
- 1 Avocado, diced

For Peanut Sauce:
- 1/4 cup Peanut butter
- 1/4 cup Coconut aminos
- 1 1/2 tbsp Lime juice
- 1/2 tsp crushed red pepper flakes
- 1/4 tsp Sea salt
- 1/4 tsp Garlic powder

For Garnish:
- Sliced green onions
- Lime wedges
- Roasted peanuts

Directions:
1. Combine two tbsp of olive oil, coconut aminos, fish sauce, red peppers, and lime juice in a bowl.
2. Add in the shrimp and stir to mix. Cover the bowl and keep it aside to marinate for thirty minutes.
3. Combine the peanut sauce ingredients and keep them aside. Pour two tbsp of oil into a pan and place over medium heat.
4. Add in shrimp and cook until opaque, about six minutes. Share the cucumbers, shrimp, and avocados among the lettuce leaves. Add in a drizzle of peanut sauce and garnish with peanuts, green onions, and lime wedges if desired.

Nutrition:
- Calories: 470
- Protein: 29 g
- Fat: 31 g
- Carbohydrates: 16 g

270. <u>Tasty Low Carb Cucumber Salad</u>

Difficulty: Easy
Preparation Time: 10 minutes
Cooking Time: 0 minutes
Servings: 6
Ingredients:
- 1/2 cup Sour cream
- 2 tbsp Fresh dill, chopped
- 1 tbsp Olive oil
- 1 tbsp Lemon juice
- 1/2 tsp Garlic powder
- 1/2 tsp Sea salt
- 1/4 tsp Black pepper
- 6 cups Cucumber, chopped
- 1 Red onion, thinly sliced

Directions:
1. Combine the dill, sour cream, olive oil, garlic powder, and lemon juice in a bowl. Season the mixture with black pepper and sea salt.
2. Add in the red onions and chopped cucumbers. Serve.

Nutrition:
- Calories: 86
- Protein: 2 g
- Fat: 6 g
- Carbohydrates: 7 g

271. Classic Low Carb Cobb Salad

Difficulty: Easy
Preparation Time: 30 minutes
Cooking Time: 10 minutes
Servings: 6
Ingredients:
- 1/4 cup red wine vinegar
- 2 tsp salt
- 1 tsp lemon juice
- 1 garlic clove, minced
- 3/4 tsp coarsely ground pepper
- 3/4 tsp Worcestershire sauce
- 1/4 tsp sugar
- 1/4 tsp ground mustard
- 3/4 cup canola oil
- 1/4 cup olive oil

For Salad:
- 6-1/2 cups torn romaine
- 2-1/2 cups torn curly endive
- 1 bunch watercress, trimmed, divided
- 2 chicken breasts, cooked, chopped
- 2 tomatoes, seeded and chopped
- 1 ripe avocado, peeled and chopped
- 3 boiled large eggs, chopped
- 1/2 cup crumbled blue or Roquefort cheese
- 6 cooked bacon strips, crumbled
- 2 tbsp minced fresh chives

Directions:
1. Puree the first eight ingredients in the blender, while adding olive and canola oils until smooth.
2. Mix the endive, romaine, and half of the watercress in a bowl. Transfer to a platter, then assemble the tomatoes, chicken, eggs, avocado, bacon, and cheese on the greens.
3. Top with chives and the rest of the watercress. Drizzle one cup of dressing over the salad and serve.

Nutrition:
- Calories: 577
- Protein: 20 g
- Fat: 52 g
- Carbohydrates: 10 g

272. Yummy Keto Mushroom Asparagus Frittata

Difficulty: Intermediate
Preparation Time: 25 minutes
Cooking Time: 20 minutes
Servings: 8
Ingredients:
- 8 eggs
- 1/2 cup whole-milk ricotta cheese
- 2 tbsp lemon juice
- 1/2 tsp salt
- 1/4 tsp pepper
- 1 tbsp olive oil
- 1 package frozen asparagus spears, thawed
- 1 onion, halved and thinly sliced
- 1/4 cup baby Portobello mushrooms, sliced
- 1/2 cup sweet green or red pepper, finely chopped

Directions:
1. First, preheat the oven to about 350°F, then whisk the ricotta cheese, eggs, salt, lemon juice, and pepper in a bowl.
2. Pour oil into a skillet and add onion, asparagus, mushrooms, and red pepper. Cook until pepper and onions are tender, about eight minutes.
3. Add in the egg mixture and transfer to the oven. Bake until eggs are set, about twenty-five minutes.
4. Keep aside to cool, then cut into wedges.

Nutrition:
- Calories: 130

- Protein: 9 g
- Fat: 8 g
- Carbohydrates: 5 g

273. **Yogurt Garlic Chicken**

Difficulty: Easy
Preparation Time: 30 minutes
Cooking Time: 60 min
Servings: 6
Ingredients:
- 6 pieces Pita bread rounds, halved
- 1 cup English cucumber, sliced thinly, w/each slice halved

Chicken & vegetables:
- 3 tbsp Olive oil
- 1/2 tsp Black pepper, freshly ground
- 20 ounces Chicken thighs, skinless, boneless
- 1-piece Bell pepper, red, sliced into half-inch portions
- 4 pieces Garlic cloves, chopped finely
- 1/2 tsp Cumin, ground
- 1-piece Red onion, medium, sliced into half-inch wedges
- 1/2 cup Yogurt, plain, Fat: free
- 2 tbsp Lemon juice
- 1 ½ tsp Salt
- 1/2 tsp Red pepper flakes, crushed
- 1/2 tsp Allspice, ground
- 1-piece Bell pepper, yellow, sliced into half-inch portions

Yogurt sauce:
- 2 tbsp Olive oil
- 1/4 tsp Salt
- 1 tbsp Parsley, flat-leaf, chopped finely
- 1 cup Yogurt, plain, Fat-free
- 1 tbsp Lemon juice, fresh
- 1-piece Garlic clove, chopped finely

Directions:
1. Mix the yogurt (1/2 cup), garlic cloves (4 pieces), olive oil (1 tbsp), salt (1 tsp), lemon juice (2 tbsp), pepper (1/4 tsp), allspice, cumin, and pepper flakes. Stir in the chicken and coat well. Cover and marinate in the fridge for two hours.
2. Preheat the air fryer to 400°F.
3. Grease a rimmed baking sheet (18x13-inch) with cooking spray.
4. Toss the bell peppers and onion with the remaining olive oil (2 tbsp), pepper (1/4 tsp), and salt (1/2 tsp).
5. Arrange veggies on the left side of the baking sheet and the marinated chicken thighs (drain first) on the right side. Cook in the air fryer for twenty-five to thirty minutes.
6. Mix the yogurt sauce ingredients.
7. Slice air-fried chicken into half-inch strips.
8. Top each pita round with chicken strips, roasted veggies, cucumbers, and yogurt sauce.

Nutrition:
- Calories: 380
- Fat: 10 g
- Protein 20 g
- Carbohydrates: 30 g

274. **Grilled Ham & Cheese**

Difficulty: Easy
Preparation Time: 15 minutes
Cooking Time: 30 minutes
Servings: 2
Ingredients:
- 3 low-carb buns
- 4 slices medium-cut deli ham
- 1 tbsp salted butter
- 1 oz. flour
- 3 slices cheddar cheese
- 3 slices muenster cheese

Directions:
Bread:
1. Preheat your fryer to 350°F/175°C.
2. Mix the flour, salt, and baking powder in a bowl. Put to the side.
3. Add the butter and coconut oil to a skillet.
4. Melt for 20 seconds and pour into another bowl.
5. In this bowl, mix in the dough.
6. Scramble two eggs. Add to the dough.
7. Add ½ tbsp of coconut flour to thicken, and place evenly into a cupcake tray. Fill about ¾ inch.

8. Bake for 20 minutes until browned.
9. Allow to cool for 15 minutes and cut each in half for the buns.

Sandwich:
1. Fry the deli meat in a skillet on high heat.
2. Put the ham and cheese between the buns.
3. Heat the butter on medium-high.
4. When brown, turn to low and add the dough to the pan.
5. Press down with weight until you smell burning, then flip to crisp both sides.
6. Enjoy!

Nutrition:
- Calories: 188
- Carbs: 12 g
- Fat: 16 g
- Protein: 14 g
- Fiber: 18 g

275. Prosciutto Spinach Salad

Difficulty: Easy
Preparation Time: 5 minutes
Cooking Time: 5 minutes
Servings: 2
Ingredients:
- 2 cups baby spinach
- 1/3 lb. prosciutto
- 1 cantaloupe
- 1 avocado
- ¼ cup diced red onion handful of raw, unsalted walnuts

Directions:
1. Put a cup of spinach on each plate.
2. Top with the diced prosciutto, cubes of balls of melon, slices of avocado, a handful of red onion, and a few walnuts.
3. Add some freshly ground pepper, if you like.
4. Serve!

Nutrition:
- Calories: 348
- Carbs: 11 g
- Fat: 9 g
- Protein: 26 g
- Fiber: 22 g

276. Riced Cauliflower & Curry Chicken

Difficulty: Intermediate
Preparation Time: 15 minutes
Cooking Time: 30 minutes
Servings: 6
Ingredients:
- 2 lb. chicken (4 breasts)
- 1 packet curry paste
- 3 tbsp ghee (can substitute with butter)
- ½ cup heavy cream
- 1 head cauliflower (around 1 kg)

Directions:
1. In a large skillet, melt the ghee.
2. Add the curry paste and mix.
3. Once combined, add a cup of water and simmer for 5 minutes.
4. Add the chicken, cover the skillet and simmer for 18 minutes.
5. Cut a cauliflower head into florets and blend in a food processor to make the riced cauliflower.
6. When the chicken is cooked, uncover, add the cream and cook for an additional 7 minutes.
7. Serve!

Nutrition:
- Calories: 267
- Carbs: 42 g
- Fat: 31 g
- Protein: 34 g
- Fiber: 32 g

277. Mashed Garlic Turnips

Difficulty: Easy
Preparation Time: 5 minutes
Cooking Time: 10 minutes
Servings: 2
Ingredients:
- 3 cups diced turnip
- 2 garlic cloves, minced
- ¼ cup heavy cream
- 3 tbsp melted butter
- Salt and pepper to season

Directions:
1. Boil the turnips until tender.
2. Drain and mash the turnips.
3. Add the cream, butter, salt, pepper, and garlic. Combine well.
4. Serve!

Nutrition:
- Calories: 488
- Carbs: 32 g
- Fat: 19 g
- Protein: 34 g
- Fiber: 20 g

278. Lasagna Spaghetti Squash

Difficulty: Easy
Preparation Time: 30 minutes
Cooking Time: 90 minutes
Servings: 6
Ingredients:
- 25 slices mozzarella cheese
- 1 large jar (40 oz.) Rao's Marinara sauce
- 30 oz. whole-milk ricotta cheese
- 2 large spaghetti squash, cooked (44 oz.)
- 4 lb. ground beef

Directions:
1. Preheat your fryer to 375°F/190°C.
2. Slice the spaghetti squash and place it face down inside a fryer-proof dish. Fill with water until covered.
3. Bake for 45 minutes until skin is soft.
4. Sear the meat until browned.
5. In a large skillet, heat the browned meat and marinara sauce. Set aside when warm.
6. Scrape the flesh off the cooked squash to resemble strands of spaghetti.
7. Layer the lasagna in a large greased pan in alternating layers of spaghetti squash, meat sauce, mozzarella, and ricotta. Repeat until all increases have been used.
8. Bake for 30 minutes and serve!

Nutrition:
- Calories: 508
- Carbs: 32 g
- Fat: 8 g
- Protein: 22 g
- Fiber: 21 g

279. Blue Cheese Chicken Wedges

Difficulty: Easy
Preparation Time: 20 minutes
Cooking Time: 45 minutes
Servings: 4
Ingredients:
- Blue cheese dressing
- 2 tbsp crumbled blue cheese
- 4 strips bacon
- 2 chicken breasts (boneless)
- 3/4 cup your favorite buffalo sauce

Directions:
1. Boil a large pot of salted water.
2. Add two chicken breasts to the pot and cook for 28 minutes.
3. Turn off the heat and let the chicken rest for 10 minutes. Using a fork, pull the chicken apart into strips.
4. Cook and cool the bacon strips and put them to the side.
5. On medium heat, combine the chicken and buffalo sauce. Stir until hot.
6. Add the blue cheese and buffalo pulled chicken. Top with the cooked bacon crumbles.
7. Serve and enjoy.

Nutrition:
- Calories: 309
- Carbs: 27 g
- Fat: 18 g
- Protein: 34 g
- Fiber: 29 g

280. 'Oh so good' Salad

Difficulty: Easy
Preparation Time: 5 minutes
Cooking Time: 10 minutes
Servings: 2
Ingredients:
- 6 Brussels sprouts
- ½ tsp apple cider vinegar
- 1 tsp olive/grapeseed oil
- 1 grind salt

- 1 tbsp freshly grated parmesan

Directions:
1. Slice the clean Brussels sprouts in half.
2. Cut thin slices in the opposite direction.
3. Once sliced, cut the roots off and discard.
4. Toss together with the apple cider, oil and salt.
5. Sprinkle with the parmesan cheese, combine and enjoy!

Nutrition:
- Calories: 438
- Carbs: 31 g
- Fat: 23 g
- Protein: 24 g
- Fiber: 16 g

281. **'I Love Bacon'**

Difficulty: Medium
Preparation Time: 35 minutes
Cooking Time: 90 minutes
Servings: 4
Ingredients:
- 30 slices thick-cut bacon
- 12 oz. steak
- 10 oz. pork sausage
- 4 oz. cheddar cheese, shredded

Directions:
1. Lay out 5 x 6 slices of bacon in a woven pattern and bake at 400°F/200°C for 20 minutes until crisp.
2. Combine the steak, bacon, and sausage to form a meaty mixture.
3. Lay out the meat in a rectangle of similar size to the bacon strips. Season with salt/pepper.
4. Place the bacon weave on top of the meat mixture.
5. Place the cheese in the center of the bacon.
6. Roll the meat into a tight roll and refrigerate.
7. Make a 7 x 7 bacon weave and roll the bacon weave over the meat, diagonally.
8. Bake at 400°F/200°C for 60 minutes or 165°F/75°C internally.
9. Let rest for 5 minutes before serving.

Nutrition:
- Calories: 190
- Carbs: 17 g
- Fat: 15 g
- Protein: 39 g
- Fiber: 53 g

282. **Lemon Dill Trout**

Difficulty: Easy
Preparation Time: 10 minutes
Cooking Time: 10 minutes
Servings: 1
Ingredients:
- 2 lb. pan-dressed trout (or other small fish), fresh or frozen
- 1 ½ tsp salt
- ½ cup butter or margarine
- 2 tbsp dill weed
- 3 tbsp lemon juice

Directions:
1. Cut the fish lengthwise and season them with pepper.
2. Prepare a skillet by melting the butter and dill weed.
3. Fry the fish on high heat, flesh side down, for 2–3 minutes per side.
4. Remove the fish. Add the lemon juice to the butter and dill to create a sauce.
5. Serve the fish with the sauce.

Nutrition:
- Calories: 367
- Carbs: 25 g
- Fat: 14 g
- Protein: 40 g
- Fiber: 21 g

283. **Meatballs Curry**

Difficulty: Easy
Preparation Time: 15 minutes
Cooking Time: 25 minutes
Servings: 6
Ingredients:
Meatballs:
- 1-pound lean ground pork
- 2 organic eggs, beaten
- 3 tbsp yellow onion, finely chopped
- ¼ cup fresh parsley leaves, chopped

- ¼ tsp fresh ginger, minced
- 2 garlic cloves, minced
- 1 jalapeño pepper, seeded and finely chopped
- 1 tsp granulated erythritol
- 1 tsp curry powder
- 3 tbsp olive oil

Curry:
- 1 yellow onion, chopped
- Salt, as required
- 2 garlic cloves, minced
- ¼ tsp fresh ginger, minced
- 1 tbsp curry powder
- 1 (14-ounce) can unsweetened coconut milk
- Ground black pepper, as required
- ¼ cup fresh parsley, minced

Directions:
For meatballs:
1. Place all the ingredients (except oil) in a large bowl and mix until well combined.
2. Make small-sized balls from the mixture.
3. Heat the oil in a large wok over medium heat and cook meatballs for about 3–5 minutes or until golden brown from all sides.
4. Transfer the meatballs into a bowl.

For curry:
1. In the same wok, add onion and a pinch of salt, and sauté for about 4–5 minutes.
2. Add the garlic and ginger, and sauté for about 1 minute.
3. Add the curry powder and sauté for about 1–2 minutes.
4. Add coconut milk and meatballs, and bring to a gentle simmer.
5. Adjust the heat to low and simmer, covered for about 10–12 minutes.
6. Season with salt and black pepper and remove from the heat.
7. Top with parsley and serve.

Nutrition: Calories 350, Fat 13, Carbs 6, Protein 16

284. <u>Pork with Veggies</u>

Difficulty: Medium
Preparation Time: 15 minutes
Cooking Time: 15 minutes
Servings: 5
Ingredients:
- 1-pound pork loin, cut into thin strips
- 2 tbsp olive oil, divided
- 1 tsp garlic, minced
- 1 tsp fresh ginger, minced
- 2 tbsp low-sodium soy sauce
- 1 tbsp fresh lemon juice
- 1 tsp sesame oil
- 1 tbsp granulated erythritol
- 1 tsp arrowroot starch
- 10 ounces broccoli florets
- 1 carrot, peeled and sliced
- 1 large red bell pepper, seeded and cut into strips
- 2 scallions, cut into 2-inch pieces

Directions:
1. In a bowl, mix well pork strips, ½ tbsp of olive oil, garlic, and ginger.
2. For the sauce: Add the soy sauce, lemon juice, sesame oil, Swerve, and arrowroot starch in a small bowl and mix well.
3. Heat the remaining olive oil in a large nonstick wok over high heat and sear the pork strips for about 3–4 minutes or until cooked through.
4. With a slotted spoon, transfer the pork into a bowl.
5. In the same wok, add the carrot and cook for about 2–3 minutes.
6. Add the broccoli, bell pepper, and scallion, and cook, covered for about 1–2 minutes.
7. Stir the cooked pork, sauce, and stir-fry, and cook for about 3–5 minutes or until the desired doneness, stirring occasionally.
8. Remove from the heat and serve.

Nutrition:
- Calories: 315
- Fat: 19 g
- Carbs: 11 g
- Protein: 27 g

285. Pork Taco Bake

Difficulty: Easy
Preparation Time: 15 minutes
Cooking Time: 1 hour
Servings: 6
Ingredients:
- 3 organic eggs
- ½ tsp taco seasoning
- 4 ounces canned chopped green chilies
- ¼ cup sugar-free tomato sauce
- 3 tsp taco seasoning
- 8 ounces cheddar cheese, shredded
- ¼ cup fresh basil leaves

Directions:
1. Preheat your oven to 375°F.
2. Lightly grease a 13x9-inch baking dish.
3. For the crust: In a bowl, add the eggs and cream cheese, and beat until well combined and smooth.
4. Add the taco seasoning and heavy cream, and mix well.
5. Place cheddar cheese evenly in the bottom of the prepared baking dish.
6. Spread the cream cheese mixture evenly over the cheese.
7. Bake for about 25–30 minutes.
8. Remove the baking dish from the oven and set aside for about 5 minutes.
9. Meanwhile, for the topping: Heat a large nonstick wok over medium-high heat and cook the pork for about 8–10 minutes.
10. Drain the excess grease from the wok.
11. Stir in the green chilies, tomato sauce, and taco seasoning, and remove from the heat.
12. Place the pork mixture evenly over the crust and sprinkle with cheese.
13. Bake for about 18–20 minutes or until bubbly.
14. Remove from the oven and set aside for about 5 minutes.
15. Cut into desired size slices and serve with the garnishing of basil leaves.

Nutrition:
- Calories: 556
- Fat: 39 g
- Carbs: 5 g
- Protein: 43 g

286. Spinach Pie

Difficulty: Easy
Preparation Time: 15 minutes
Cooking Time: 38 minutes
Servings: 5
Ingredients:
- 2 tbsp butter, divided
- 2 tbsp yellow onion, chopped
- 1 (16-ounce) bag frozen chopped spinach, thawed and squeezed
- 1½ cup heavy cream
- 3 organic eggs
- ½ tsp ground nutmeg
- Salt and ground black pepper, as required
- ½ cup Swiss cheese, shredded

Directions:
1. Preheat your oven to 375°F.
2. Grease a 9-inch baking dish.
3. In a large wok, melt 1 tbsp of butter over medium-high heat and sauté onion for about 4–5 minutes.
4. Add spinach and cook for about 2–3 minutes or until all the liquid is absorbed.
5. In a bowl, add cream, eggs, nutmeg, salt, and black pepper, and beat until well combined.
6. Transfer the spinach mixture to the bottom of the prepared baking dish evenly.
7. Place the egg mixture over the spinach mixture evenly and sprinkle with cheese.
8. Top with the remaining butter in the shape of dots in many places.
9. Bake for about 25–30 minutes or until the top becomes golden brown.

Nutrition:
- Calories: 267
- Fat: 9 g
- Carbs: 1 g
- Protein: 24 g

287. Baked Chicken Fajitas

Difficulty: Easy
Preparation Time: 10 minutes
Cooking Time: 18 minutes
Servings: 6
Ingredients:
- 1 1/2 lb. chicken tenders
- 2 tbsp fajita seasoning
- 2 tbsp olive oil
- 1 onion, sliced
- 2 bell pepper, sliced
- 1 lime juice
- 1 tsp kosher salt

Directions:
1. Preheat the oven to 400°F.
2. Add all the ingredients to a large mixing bowl and toss well.
3. Transfer the bowl mixture to a baking tray and bake in preheated oven for 15–18 minutes.
4. Serve and enjoy.

Nutrition:
- Calories: 286
- Fat: 13 g
- Carbs: 7 g
- Protein: 33 g

288. Pesto Zucchini Noodles

Difficulty: Easy
Preparation Time: 5 Minutes
Cooking Time: 2 Minutes
Servings: 4
Ingredients:
- 3 lb. Zucchini
- Spiral Slicer
- Olive Oil

Directions:
1. Prepare the Zucchini: trim the ends away from your zucchini.
2. Using the instructions for your spiral slicer, slice the zucchini into noodles.
3. Store, Or Cook: Simply heat a saucepan with olive oil over medium heat. Sauté zoodles for 5 minutes, until tender!

Nutrition:
- Calories: 56
- Fat: 1 g
- Carbs: 11 g
- Protein: 2 g

289. Sautéed Crispy Zucchini

Difficulty: Medium
Preparation Time: 15 minutes
Cooking Time: 38 minutes
Servings: 5
Ingredients:
- 2 tbsp butter
- 4 zucchinis, cut into 1/4-in.-thick rounds
- 1/4 cup freshly grated Parmesan cheese
- Freshly ground black pepper

Directions:
1. In a large skillet over medium-high heat, melt butter.
2. Add zucchini and cook, stirring occasionally, until tender and lightly browned, about 5 min.
3. Spread zucchini evenly in skillet and sprinkle Parmesan over vegetables.
4. Cook without stirring until Parmesan is melted and crispy where it touches the skillet for about 5 min. Top with pepper and serve.

Nutrition:
- Calories: 156
- Fat: 4 g
- Carbs: 0 g
- Protein: 2 g

DINNER RECIPES

290. Zucchini Salmon Salad

Difficulty: Easy
Preparation Time: 5 minutes
Cooking Time: 10 minutes
Servings: 3
Ingredients:
- 2 salmon fillets
- 2 tbsp soy sauce
- 2 zucchinis, sliced
- Salt and pepper to taste
- 2 tbsp extra virgin olive oil
- 2 tbsp sesame seeds
- Salt and pepper to taste

Directions:
1. Drizzle the salmon with soy sauce.
2. Heat a grill pan over a medium flame. Cook salmon on the grill on each side for 2–3 minutes.
3. Season the zucchini with salt and pepper and place it on the grill as well. Cook on each side until golden.
4. Place the zucchini, salmon, and the rest of the ingredients in a bowl.
5. Serve the salad fresh.

Nutrition:
- Calories: 224
- Fat: 19 g
- Protein: 18 g
- Carbohydrates: 0 g

291. Pan Fried Salmon

Difficulty: Easy
Preparation Time: 5 minutes
Cooking Time: 20 minutes
Servings: 4
Ingredients:
- 4 salmon fillets
- Salt and pepper to taste
- 1 tsp dried oregano
- 1 tsp dried basil
- 3 tbsp extra virgin olive oil

Directions:
1. Season the fish with salt, pepper, oregano, and basil.
2. Heat the oil in a pan and place the salmon in the hot oil, with the skin facing down.
3. Fry on each side for 2 minutes until golden brown and fragrant.
4. Serve the salmon warm and fresh.

Nutrition:
- Calories: 327
- Fat: 25 g
- Protein: 36 g
- Carbs: 0.3 g

292. Grilled Salmon with Pineapple Salsa

Difficulty: Intermediate
Preparation Time: 5 minutes
Cooking Time: 30 minutes
Servings: 4
Ingredients:
- 4 salmon fillets
- Salt and pepper to taste
- 2 tbsp Cajun seasoning
- 1 fresh pineapple, peeled and diced
- 1 cup cherry tomatoes, quartered
- 2 tbsp cilantro, chopped
- 2 tbsp parsley, chopped
- 1 tsp mint, dried
- 2 tbsp lemon juice
- 2 tbsp extra virgin olive oil
- 1 tsp honey
- Salt and pepper to taste

Directions:
1. Add salt, pepper, and Cajun seasoning to the fish.
2. Heat a grill pan over a medium flame. Cook fish on the grill on each side for 3–4 minutes.
3. For the salsa, mix the pineapple, tomatoes, cilantro, parsley, mint, lemon juice, olive oil,

and honey in a bowl. Season with salt and pepper.
4. Serve the grilled salmon with the pineapple salsa.

Nutrition:
- Calories: 332
- Fat: 12 g
- Protein: 34 g
- Carbs: 0 g

293. Mediterranean Chickpea Salad

Difficulty: Easy
Preparation Time: 5 minutes
Cooking Time: 20 minutes
Servings: 6
Ingredients:
- 1 can chickpeas, drained
- 1 fennel bulb, sliced
- 1 red onion, sliced
- 1 tsp basil, dried
- 1 tsp oregano, dried
- 2 tbsp parsley, chopped
- 4 garlic cloves, minced
- 2 tbsp lemon juice
- 2 tbsp extra virgin olive oil
- Salt and pepper to taste

Directions:
1. Combine the chickpeas, fennel, red onion, herbs, garlic, lemon juice, and oil in a salad bowl.
2. Add salt and pepper and serve the salad fresh.

Nutrition:
- Calories: 200
- Fat: 9 g
- Protein: 4 g
- Carbs: 28 g

294. Warm Chorizo Chickpea Salad

Difficulty: Easy
Preparation Time: 5 minutes
Cooking Time: 20 minutes
Servings: 6
Ingredients:
- 1 tbsp extra-virgin olive oil
- 4 chorizo links, sliced
- 1 red onion, sliced
- 4 red bell peppers, chopped, roasted
- 1 can chickpeas, drained
- 2 cups cherry tomatoes
- 2 tbsp balsamic vinegar
- Salt and pepper to taste

Directions:
1. Heat the oil in a skillet and add the chorizo. Cook briefly just until fragrant, then add the onion, bell peppers, and chickpeas and cook for 2 additional minutes.
2. Transfer the mixture to a salad bowl, then add the tomatoes, vinegar, salt, and pepper.
3. Mix well and serve the salad right away.

Nutrition:
- Calories: 359
- Fat: 18 g
- Protein: 15 g
- Carbs: 21 g

295. Jalapeno Lentil Burgers

Difficulty: Easy
Preparation Time: 15 minutes
Cooking Time: 10 minutes
Servings: 5
Ingredients:
- 1/2 cup dried red lentils; rinsed
- 1–12 oz. can chickpeas; rinsed
- 1 tsp ground cumin;
- 1 tsp chili powder
- 1 tsp sea salt
- 1/2 cup packed cilantro
- 2 Garlic cloves, minced
- 4 Jalapeno, finely chopped
- 1/2 small red onion; minced
- 1 Red bell pepper
- 2 Carrot; shredded
- 1/4 cup oat bran/oat flour; (gluten-free)
- Lettuce for serving
- 5 Hamburger buns

- 2 cups water
- 2 tbsp olive oil (optional)

For pico:
- 1 ripe mango, diced
- 1 ripe avocado, diced
- 1/2 small red onion; finely diced
- 1/2 cup cilantro; chopped
- 1/2 tsp fresh lime juice
- Sea salt

Directions:
1. Put all the ingredients in a large bowl and mix.
2. Stir in the salt to compare.
3. Put a medium saucepan on medium heat, add lentils plus 1 1/2 cups of water, then bring water to a boil, cover it afterward, lower the heat to low, and then simmer lentils until the water is absorbed.
4. Drain, and set aside some extra water.
5. In a food processor, put the cooked lentils, chickpeas, garlic, sea salt, cilantro, chili powder, and cumin, and blend until the beans and lentils are smooth.
6. Add tomato, red pepper, jalapeno, and carrot to compare.
7. Divide into 6 equal parts and use your hands to create dense patties.
8. Heat skillet over a medium-high flame; apply 1/2 tbsp of olive oil.
9. Place a few burgers in at a time and cook on either side for a couple of minutes, just until crisp and golden brown.
10. Repeat with the remaining patties and add olive oil whenever desired.
11. Place the patties in a bun or lettuce and finish with mango avocado pico.

Nutrition:
- Carbs: 34.9 g
- Calories: 225
- Sugar: 7.7 g
- Fats: 6.1 g

296. Grandma's Rice

Difficulty: Easy
Preparation Time: 15 minutes
Cooking Time: 2 hours
Servings: 4
Ingredients:
- 40 g butter
- 1/2 cup brown sugar
- 1/2 cup Arborio rice
- 3 cups milk
- 1/2 tbsp ground cinnamon
- 1/8 tbsp ground nutmeg
- 1 tbsp vanilla paste
- 1/2 cup raisins
- 300 ml. cream

Directions:
1. Preheat the oven to 300°F.
2. Grease a 1-liter ability oven-safe plate.
3. Heat butter in a saucepan and add sugar and rice.
4. Stir for 1 minute to thoroughly coat the rice.
5. Remove from heat and whisk in milk, spices, and vanilla.
6. Stir through raisins, then pour into the prepared plate.
7. Bake for 30 minutes, then remove from the oven and stir well.
8. Drizzle over the cream and return to the oven for an additional hour.
9. Check that the rice is cooked through.
10. Return to the oven for 15–30 minutes if required.
11. Serve with extra cream and nutmeg.

Nutrition:
- Fat: 20 g
- Protein: 23 g
- Cholesterol: 25 mg
- Carbs: 30 g
- Sodium: 1000 mg.

297. Baked Beef Zucchini

Difficulty: Medium
Preparation Time: 10 minutes
Cooking Time: 40 minutes
Servings: 4
Ingredients:
- 2 large zucchinis
- 1 cup beef, minced
- 1 cup mushroom, chopped
- 1 tomato, chopped
- 1/2 cup spinach, chopped
- 1 tbsp chives, minced
- 2 tbsp olive oil
- Salt and pepper to taste
- 1 tbsp almond butter
- 1 tsp garlic powder
- 1 cup Cheddar cheese, grated
- 1/3 tsp ginger powder

Directions:
1. Preheat the oven to 400°F.
2. Add aluminum foil to a baking sheet.
3. Cut the zucchini in half. Scoop out the seeds and make pockets to stuff them later.
4. In a pan, add the olive oil.
5. Toss the beef until brown.
6. Add the mushroom, tomato, chives, salt, pepper, garlic, ginger, and spinach.
7. Cook for 2 minutes. Take off the heat.
8. Stuff the zucchinis using the mix.
9. Add them to the baking sheet. Sprinkle the cheese on top.
10. Add the butter on top. Bake for 30 minutes. Serve warm.

Nutrition:
- Fat: 12.8 g
- Cholesterol: 79.7 mg
- Sodium: 615.4 mg
- Potassium: 925.8 mg
- Carbs: 26.8 g

298. Baked Tuna with Asparagus

Difficulty: Easy
Preparation Time: 10 minutes
Cooking Time: 10 minutes
Servings: 2
Ingredients:
- 2 tuna steak
- 1 cup asparagus, trimmed
- 1 tsp almond butter
- 1 tsp rosemary
- 1/2 tsp oregano
- 1/2 tsp garlic powder
- 1 tsp lemon juice
- 1/2 tsp ginger powder
- 1 tbsp olive oil
- 1 tsp red chili powder
- Salt and pepper to taste

Directions:
1. Marinate the tuna using oregano, lemon juice, salt, pepper, red chili powder, garlic, ginger, and let it sit for 10 minutes.
2. In a pan, add the olive oil.
3. Fry the tuna steaks for 2 minutes per side.
4. In another pan, melt the almond butter.
5. Toss the asparagus with salt, pepper, and rosemary for 3 minutes.
6. Serve.

Nutrition:
- Fat: 4.7 g
- Cholesterol: 0 mg
- Sodium: 98.5 mg
- Potassium: 171.6 mg
- Carbs: 3.2 g

299. Lamb Stuffed Avocado

Difficulty: Easy
Preparation Time: 10 minutes
Cooking Time: 40 minutes
Servings: 4
Ingredients:
- 2 avocados
- 1 1/2 cup lamb, minced
- 1/2 cup Cheddar cheese, grated
- 1/2 cup Parmesan cheese, grated
- 2 tbsp almond, chopped
- 1 tbsp coriander, chopped
- 2 tbsp olive oil
- 1 tomato, chopped
- 1 jalapeno, chopped
- Salt and pepper to taste
- 1 tsp garlic, chopped
- 1-inch ginger, chopped

Directions:
1. Cut the avocados in half. Remove the pit and scoop out some flesh to stuff it later.
2. In a skillet, add half of the oil.
3. Toss the ginger, garlic for 1 minute.
4. Add the lamb and toss for 3 minutes.
5. Add the tomato, coriander, parmesan, jalapeno, salt, pepper, and cook for 2 minutes.
6. Take off the heat. Stuff the avocados.
7. Sprinkle the almonds, Cheddar cheese, and add olive oil on top.
8. Add to a baking sheet and bake for 30 minutes. Serve.

Nutrition:
- Fat: 19.5 g
- Cholesterol: 167.5 mg
- Sodium: 410.7 mg
- Potassium: 617.1 mg
- Carbs: 13.1 g

300. Mozzarella Sticks

Difficulty: Easy
Preparation Time: 8 minutes
Cooking Time: 2 minutes
Servings: 2
Ingredients:
- 1 large whole egg
- 3 sticks Mozzarella cheese in half (frozen overnight)
- 2 tbsp Parmesan cheese, grated
- 1/2 cup almond flour
- 1/4 cup coconut oil
- 2 1/2 tsp Italian seasoning blend
- 1 tbsp parsley, chopped
- 1/2 tsp salt
- ½ cup keto marinara sauce (optional)

Directions:
1. Heat the coconut oil in a cast-iron skillet of medium size over low-medium heat.
2. Crack the egg in a small bowl in the meantime and beat it well.
3. Take another bowl of medium size and add Parmesan cheese, almond flour, and seasonings to it. Whisk together the ingredients until a smooth mixture is prepared.
4. Take the overnight frozen Mozzarella stick and dip it in the beaten egg, then coat it well with the dry mixture. Do the same with all the remaining cheese sticks.
5. Place all the coated sticks in the preheated skillet and cook them for 2 minutes or until they start giving a golden-brown look from all sides.
6. Remove from the skillet once cooked properly and place over a paper towel so that any extra oil gets absorbed.
7. Sprinkle parsley over the sticks, if you desire, and serve with keto marinara sauce.

Nutrition:
- Calories: 430
- Fat: 39 g
- Carbohydrates: 10 g
- Protein: 20 g

301. Greek Roasted Fish

Difficulty: Easy
Preparation Time: 5 minutes
Cooking Time: 30 minutes
Servings: 4
Ingredients:
- 4 salmon fillets
- 1 tbsp chopped oregano
- 1 tsp dried basil
- 1 zucchini, sliced
- 1 red onion, sliced
- 1 carrot, sliced
- 1 lemon, sliced
- 2 tbsp extra virgin olive oil
- Salt and pepper to taste

Directions:
1. Add all the ingredients to a deep dish baking skillet.
2. Season with salt and pepper and cook in the preheated oven at 350°F for 20 minutes.
3. Serve the fish and vegetables warm.

Nutrition:
- Calories: 328
- Fat: 13 g
- Carbs: 2 g
- Protein: 38 g

302. Tomato Fish Bake

Difficulty: Easy
Preparation Time: 5 minutes
Cooking Time: 30 minutes
Servings: 4
Ingredients:
- 4 cod fillets
- 4 tomatoes, sliced
- 4 garlic cloves, minced
- 1 shallot, sliced
- 1 celery stalk, sliced
- 1 tsp fennel seeds
- 1 cup vegetable stock
- Salt and pepper to taste

Directions:
1. Layer the cod fillets and tomatoes in a deep dish baking skillet.
2. Add the rest of the ingredients and add salt and pepper.
3. Cook in the oven at 350°F for 20 minutes.
4. Serve the dish warm or chilled.

Nutrition:
- Calories: 299
- Fat: 3 g
- Carbs: 3 g
- Protein: 64 g

303. Garlicky Tomato Chicken Casserole

Difficulty: Intermediate
Preparation Time: 5 minutes
Cooking Time: 30 minutes
Servings: 4
Ingredients:
- 4 chicken breasts
- 2 tomatoes, sliced
- 1 can diced tomatoes
- 2 garlic cloves, chopped
- 1 shallot, chopped
- 1 bay leaf
- 1 thyme sprig
- ½ cup dry white wine
- ½ cup chicken stock
- Salt and pepper to taste

Directions:
1. Combine the chicken and the remaining ingredients in a deep dish baking skillet.
2. Adjust the taste with salt and pepper and cover the pot with a lid or aluminum foil.
3. Cook in the preheated oven at 330°F for 40 minutes.
4. Serve the casserole warm.

Nutrition:
- Calories: 313
- Fat: 8 g
- Carbs: 5 g
- Protein: 47 g

304. Chicken Cacciatore

Difficulty: Easy
Preparation Time: 5 minutes
Cooking Time: 45 minutes
Servings: 6
Ingredients:
- 2 tbsp extra virgin olive oil
- 6 chicken thighs
- 1 sweet onion, chopped
- 2 garlic cloves, minced
- 2 red bell peppers, cored and diced
- 2 carrots, diced
- 1 rosemary sprig
- 1 thyme sprig
- 4 tomatoes, peeled and diced
- ½ cup tomato juice
- ¼ cup dry white wine
- 1 cup chicken stock
- 1 bay leaf
- Salt and pepper to taste

Directions:
1. Heat the oil in a heavy saucepan.
2. Cook chicken on all sides until golden.
3. Add the mixture of garlic and onion and cook for 2 minutes.
4. Stir in the rest of the ingredients and season with salt and pepper.
5. Cook on low heat for 30 minutes.
6. Serve the chicken cacciatore warm and fresh.

Nutrition:
- Calories: 363
- Fat: 14 g
- Carbs: 7 g
- Protein: 42 g

305. Fennel Wild Rice Risotto

Difficulty: Easy
Preparation Time: 5 minutes
Cooking Time: 35 minutes
Servings: 6
Ingredients:
- 2 tbsp extra virgin olive oil
- 1 shallot, chopped
- 2 garlic cloves, minced
- 1 fennel bulb, chopped
- 1 cup wild rice
- ¼ cup dry white wine
- 2 cups chicken stock
- 1 tsp grated orange zest
- Salt and pepper to taste

Directions:
1. Heat the oil in a heavy saucepan.
2. Add the garlic, shallot, and fennel and cook for a few minutes until softened.
3. Add the rice and cook for 2 additional minutes then add the wine, stock, and orange zest, with salt and pepper to taste.
4. Cook on low heat for 20 minutes.
5. Serve the risotto warm and fresh.

Nutrition:
- Calories: 162
- Fat: 2 g
- Carbs: 5 g
- Protein: 8 g

306. Wild Rice Prawn Salad

Difficulty: Medium
Preparation Time: 5 minutes
Cooking Time: 35 minutes
Servings: 6
Ingredients:
- ¾ cup wild rice
- 1¾ cups chicken stock
- 1 pound prawns
- Salt and pepper to taste
- 2 tbsp lemon juice
- 2 tbsp extra virgin olive oil
- 2 cups arugula

Directions:
1. Combine the rice and chicken stock in a saucepan and cook until the liquid has been absorbed entirely.
2. Transfer the rice to a salad container.
3. Season the prawns with pepper and salt and sprinkle them with lemon juice and oil.
4. Heat a grill skillet over medium flame.
5. Place the prawns on the hot skillet and cook on each side for 2-3 minutes.

6. For the salad, combine the rice with arugula and prawns and mix well.
7. Serve the salad fresh.

Nutrition:
- Calories: 207
- Fat: 4 g
- Carbs: 2 g
- Protein: 20 g

307. Chicken Broccoli Salad with Avocado Dressing

Difficulty: Intermediate
Preparation Time: 5 minutes
Cooking Time: 40 minutes
Servings: 6
Ingredients:
- 2 chicken breasts
- 1-pound broccoli, cut into florets
- 1 avocado, peeled and pitted
- ½ lemon, juiced
- 2 garlic cloves
- ¼ tsp chili powder
- ¼ tsp cumin powder
- Salt and pepper to taste

Directions:
1. Cook the chicken in a large pot of salty water.
2. Drain and cut the chicken into small cubes. Place in a salad container.
3. Add the broccoli and mix well.
4. Combine the avocado, lemon juice, garlic, chili powder, cumin powder, salt, and pepper in a blender. Pulse until smooth.
5. Spread the dressing on the salad and mix well.
6. Serve the salad fresh.

Nutrition:
- Calories: 195
- Fat: 11 g
- Carbs: 12 g
- Protein: 3 g

308. Seafood Paella

Difficulty: Easy
Preparation Time: 5 minutes
Cooking Time: 40 minutes
Servings: 8
Ingredients:
- 2 tbsp extra virgin olive oil
- 1 shallot, chopped
- 2 garlic cloves, chopped
- 1 red bell pepper, cored and diced
- 1 carrot, diced
- 2 tomatoes, peeled and diced
- 1 cup wild rice
- 1 cup tomato juice
- 2 cups chicken stock
- 1 chicken breast, cubed
- Salt and pepper to taste
- 2 monkfish fillets, cubed
- ½ pound fresh shrimps, peeled and deveined
- ½ pound prawns
- 1 thyme sprig
- 1 rosemary sprig

Directions:
1. Heat the fresh oil in a skillet and stir in the shallot, garlic, bell pepper, carrot, and tomatoes. Cook for a few minutes until softened.
2. Stir in the rice, tomato juice, stock, chicken, salt, and pepper, and cook on low heat for 20 minutes.
3. Mix the remaining ingredients and cook for 10 additional minutes.
4. Serve the paella warm and fresh.

Nutrition:
- Calories: 245
- Fat: 8 g
- Carbs: 3 g
- Protein: 27 g

151. Herbed Roasted Chicken Breasts

Difficulty: Easy
Preparation Time: 5 minutes
Cooking Time: 40 minutes
Servings: 4
Ingredients:
- 2 tbsp extra virgin olive oil
- 2 tbsp chopped parsley
- 2 tbsp chopped cilantro
- 1 tsp dried oregano
- 1 tsp dried basil
- 2 tbsp lemon juice
- Salt and pepper to taste
- 4 chicken breasts

Directions:
1. Combine the oil, parsley, cilantro, oregano, basil, lemon juice, salt, and pepper in a container.
2. Spread this mixture over the chicken and rub it well into the meat.
3. Place in a deep dish baking skillet and cover with aluminum foil.
4. Cook in the oven at 350°F for 20 minutes then remove the foil and cook for 20 additional minutes.
5. Serve the chicken warm and fresh with your favorite side dish.

Nutrition:
- Calories: 330
- Fat: 14 g
- Carbs: 12 g
- Protein: 43 g

152. Marinated Chicken Breasts

Difficulty: Easy
Preparation Time: 5 minutes
Cooking Time: 20 minutes
Servings: 4
Ingredients:
- 4 chicken breasts
- Salt and pepper to taste
- 1 lemon, juiced
- 1 rosemary sprig
- 1 thyme sprig
- 2 garlic cloves, crushed
- 2 sage leaves
- 3 tbsp extra virgin olive oil
- ½ cup buttermilk

Directions:
1. Boil the chicken with salt and pepper and place it in a resealable bag.
2. Add the remaining ingredients and seal the bag.
3. Refrigerate for at least 1 hour.
4. After 1 hour, heat a roasting skillet over medium heat, then place the chicken on the grill.
5. Cook on both sides for 8–10 minutes or until juices are gone.
6. Serve the chicken warm with your favorite side dish.

Nutrition:
- Calories: 371
- Fat: 21 g
- Carbs: 2 g
- Protein: 46 g

153. Greek Style Quesadillas

Difficulty: Easy
Preparation Time: 10 minutes
Cooking Time: 10 minutes
Servings: 4
Ingredients:
- 4 whole-wheat tortillas
- 1 cup Mozzarella cheese, shredded
- 1 cup fresh spinach, chopped
- 2 tbsp Greek yogurt
- 1 egg g beaten
- ¼ cup green olives, sliced
- 1 tbsp olive oil
- 1/3 cup fresh cilantro, chopped

Directions:
1. In the container, combine together Mozzarella cheese, spinach, yogurt, egg, olives, and cilantro.
2. Then pour olive oil into the skillet.
3. Place 1 tortilla into the skillet and spread it with the Mozzarella mixture.
4. Top it with the second tortilla and spread it with the cheese mixture again.
5. Then place the third tortilla and spread it with all the remaining cheese mixture.

6. Cover it with the last tortilla and fry it for 5 minutes from each side over medium heat.

Nutrition:
- Calories: 193
- Fat: 7.7 g
- Carbs: 20 g
- Protein: 8.3 g

309. Creamy Penne

Difficulty: Easy
Preparation Time: 10 minutes
Cooking Time: 25 minutes
Servings: 4
Ingredients:
- ½ cup penne, dried
- 9 oz. chicken filet
- 1 tsp Italian seasoning
- 1 tbsp olive oil
- 1 tomato, chopped
- 1 cup heavy cream
- 1 tbsp fresh basil, chopped
- ½ tsp salt
- 2 oz. Parmesan, grated
- 1 cup water, for cooking

Directions:
1. Pour water into the skillet, add penne, and boil it for 15 minutes. Then drain the water.
2. Pour olive oil into the skillet and heat it up.
3. Slice the chicken filet and put it in the hot oil.
4. Sprinkle chicken with Italian seasoning and roast for 2 minutes from each side.
5. Then add fresh basil, salt, tomato, and grated cheese.
6. Stir well.
7. Add heavy cream and cooked penne.
8. Cook for 5 minutes more over medium heat. Stir it from time to time.

Nutrition:
- Calories: 388
- Fat: 24 g
- Carbs: 17.6 g
- Protein: 17 g

310. Light Paprika Moussaka

Difficulty: Easy
Preparation Time: 15 minutes
Cooking Time: 40 minutes
Servings: 3
Ingredients:
- 1 eggplant, trimmed
- 1 cup ground chicken
- 1/3 cup white onion, diced
- 3 oz. Cheddar cheese, shredded
- 1 potato, sliced
- 1 tsp olive oil
- 1 tsp salt
- ½ cup milk
- 1 tbsp butter
- 1 tbsp ground paprika
- 1 tbsp Italian seasoning
- 1 tsp tomato paste

Directions:
1. Cut the eggplant lengthwise and season with salt.
2. Pour olive oil into the skillet and add sliced potato.
3. Roast potatoes for 2 minutes from each side.
4. Then transfer it to the plate.
5. Put eggplant in the skillet and roast it for 2 minutes from each side too.
6. Pour milk into the skillet and bring it to a boil.
7. Add tomato paste, Italian seasoning, paprika, butter, and Cheddar cheese.
8. Then mix up the onion with ground chicken.
9. Arrange the sliced potato in the casserole in one layer.
10. Then add ½ part of all sliced eggplants.
11. Spread the eggplants with ½ part of the chicken mixture.
12. Then add the remaining eggplants.
13. Pour the milk mixture over the eggplants.
14. Bake moussaka for 30 minutes at 355°F.

Nutrition:
- Calories: 387
- Fat: 24 g
- Carbs: 22 g
- Protein: 25 g

311. Cucumber Container with Spices and Greek Yogurt

Difficulty: Intermediate
Preparation Time: 10 minutes
Cooking Time: 20 minutes
Servings: 3
Ingredients:
- 4 cucumbers
- ½ tsp chili pepper
- ¼ cup fresh parsley, chopped
- ¾ cup fresh dill, chopped
- 2 tbsp lemon juice
- ½ tsp salt
- ½ tsp ground black pepper
- ¼ tsp sage & ½ tsp dried oregano
- 1/3 cup Greek yogurt

Directions:
1. Make the cucumber dressing: blend the dill and parsley until you get green mash.
2. Then combine together green mash with lemon juice, salt, ground black pepper, sage, dried oregano, Greek yogurt, and chili pepper.
3. Churn the mixture well.
4. Chop the cucumbers roughly and combine them with cucumber dressing. Mix up well.
5. Refrigerate the cucumber for 20 minutes.

Nutrition:
- Calories: 114
- Fat: 1.6 g
- Carbs: 20 g
- Protein: 7.6 g

312. Stuffed Bell Peppers with Quinoa

Difficulty: Easy
Preparation Time: 10 minutes
Cooking Time: 35 minutes
Servings: 2
Ingredients:
- 2 bell peppers
- 1/3 cup quinoa
- 3 oz. chicken stock
- ¼ cup onion, diced
- ½ tsp salt
- ¼ tsp tomato paste
- ½ tsp dried oregano
- 1/3 cup sour cream
- 1 tsp paprika

Directions:
1. Trim the bell peppers and remove the seeds.
2. Then combine together chicken stock and quinoa in the skillet.
3. Add salt and boil the ingredients for 10 minutes or until quinoa will soak all liquid.
4. Then combine together cooked quinoa with dried oregano, tomato paste, and onion.
5. Fill the bell peppers with the quinoa combo and arrange them in the casserole mold.
6. Add sour cream and bake the peppers for 25 minutes at 365°F.
7. Serve the cooked peppers with sour cream sauce from the casserole mold.

Nutrition:
- Calories: 237
- Fat: 10.3 g
- Carbs: 22 g
- Protein: 6.3 g

313. Mediterranean Burrito

Difficulty: Easy
Preparation Time: 10 minutes
Cooking Time: 0 minutes
Servings: 2
Ingredients:
- 2 wheat tortillas
- 2 oz. red kidney beans, canned, drained
- 2 tbsp hummus
- 2 tsp tahini sauce
- 1 cucumber
- 2 lettuce leaves
- 1 tbsp lime juice
- 1 tsp olive oil
- ½ tsp dried oregano

Directions:
1. Mash the red kidney beans until you get a puree.
2. Then spread the wheat tortillas with bean mash from one side.
3. Add hummus and tahini sauce.
4. Cut the cucumber into the wedges and place them over tahini sauce.
5. Then add lettuce leaves.

6. Make the dressing: mix up together olive oil, dried oregano, and lime juice.
7. Sprinkle the lettuce leaves with the dressing and wrap the wheat tortillas in the shape of burritos.

Nutrition:
- Calories: 288
- Fat: 10.4 g
- Carbs: 18.2 g
- Protein: 13 g

314. Sweet Potato Bacon Mash

Difficulty: Intermediate
Preparation Time: 10 minutes
Cooking Time: 20 minutes
Servings: 4
Ingredients:
- 3 sweet potatoes, peeled
- 4 oz. bacon, chopped
- 1 cup chicken stock
- 1 tbsp butter
- 1 tsp salt
- 2 oz. Parmesan, grated

Directions:
1. Cut sweet potato and place it in the skillet.
2. Add chicken stock and close the lid.
3. Boil the vegetables until they are soft.
4. After this, drain the chicken stock.
5. Crush the sweet potato with the aid of the potato masher. Add grated cheese and butter.
6. Mix up together salt and chopped bacon. Fry the mixture until it is crunchy (10–15 minutes).
7. Add cooked bacon to the mashed sweet potato and mix up with the help of the spoon.
8. It is recommended to serve the meal warm or hot.

Nutrition:
- Calories: 304
- Fat: 18.1 g
- Carbs: 18.2 g
- Protein: 17 g

315. Prosciutto Wrapped Mozzarella Balls

Difficulty: Medium
Preparation Time: 10 minutes
Cooking Time: 10 minutes
Servings: 4
Ingredients:
- 8 Mozzarella balls, cherry size
- 4 oz. bacon, sliced
- ¼ tsp ground black pepper
- ¾ tsp dried rosemary
- 1 tsp butter

Directions:
1. Sprinkle the sliced bacon with ground black pepper and dried rosemary.
2. Wrap every Mozzarella ball in the sliced bacon and secure them with toothpicks.
3. Melt butter.
4. Brush the wrapped Mozzarella balls with butter.
5. Line the tray with the baking paper and arrange Mozzarella balls in it.
6. Bake the meal for 10 minutes at 365°F.

Nutrition:
- Calories: 322
- Fat: 26.8 g
- Carbs: 0.6 g
- Protein: 20.6 g

316. Garlic Chicken Balls

Difficulty: Easy
Preparation Time: 15 minutes
Cooking Time: 10 minutes
Servings: 4
Ingredients:
- 2 cups ground chicken
- 1 tsp minced garlic
- 1 tsp dried dill
- 1/3 carrot, grated
- 1 egg, beaten
- 1 tbsp olive oil
- ¼ cup coconut flakes
- ½ tsp salt

Directions:
1. In the mixing container mix up together ground chicken, minced garlic, dried dill, carrot, egg, and salt.
2. Stir the chicken mixture with the help of the fingertips until homogenous.
3. Then make medium balls from the mixture.
4. Coat every chicken ball in coconut flakes.
5. Heat up olive oil in the skillet.
6. Add chicken balls and cook them for 3 minutes from each side. The cooked chicken balls will have a golden-brown color.

Nutrition:
- Calories: 200
- Fat: 11.5 g
- Carbs: 1.7 g
- Protein: 21.3 g

317. Monkey Salad

Difficulty: Easy
Preparation Time: 4 minutes
Cooking Time: 7 minutes
Servings: 1
Ingredients:
- 2 tbsp butter
- 1 cup unsweetened coconut flakes
- 1 cup raw, unsalted cashews
- 1 cup raw, unsalted s
- 1 cup 90% dark chocolate shavings

Directions:
1. In a skillet, melt the butter on medium heat.
2. Add the coconut flakes and sauté until lightly browned for 4 minutes.
3. Add the cashews and s and sauté for 3 minutes. Remove from the heat and sprinkle with dark chocolate shavings.
4. Serve!

Nutrition:
- Calories: 321
- Fat: 12 g
- Carbs: 12 g
- Protein: 6 g

318. Jarlsberg Lunch Omelet

Difficulty: Easy
Preparation Time: 5 minutes
Cooking Time: 10 minutes
Servings: 2
Ingredients:
- 4 medium mushrooms, sliced, 2 oz.
- 1 green onion, sliced
- 2 eggs, beaten
- 1 oz. Jarlsberg or Swiss cheese, shredded
- 1 oz. ham, diced

Directions:
1. In a skillet, cook the mushrooms and green onion until tender.
2. Add the eggs and mix well.
3. Sprinkle it with salt and top with the mushroom mixture, cheese, and ham.
4. When the egg is set, fold the plain side of the omelet on the filled side.
5. Remove the heat and let it stand until the cheese has melted.
6. Serve!

Nutrition:
- Calories: 288
- Fat: 12 g
- Carbs: 22 g
- Protein: 26 g

319. Fiery Jalapeno Poppers

Difficulty: Easy
Preparation Time: 10 minutes
Cooking Time: 40 minutes
Servings: 4
Ingredients:
- 5 oz. cream cheese
- ¼ cup mozzarella cheese
- 8 medium jalapeno peppers
- ½ tsp Mrs. Dash Table Blend
- 8 slices bacon

Directions:
1. Preheat your fryer to 400°F/200°C.
2. Cut the jalapenos in half.
3. Use a spoon to pickle out the insides of the peppers.

4. In a container, add together the cream cheese, mozzarella cheese, and spices of your choice.
5. Pack the cream cheese mixture into the jalapenos and place the peppers on top.
6. Wrap every pepper in one slice of bacon, starting from the bottom and working up.
7. Bake for 30 minutes. Broil for an additional 3 minutes.
8. Serve!

Nutrition:
- Calories: 238
- Fat: 10 g
- Carbs: 4 g
- Protein: 24 g

320. Bacon & Chicken Patties

Difficulty: Easy
Preparation Time: 5 minutes
Cooking Time: 15 minutes
Servings: 2
Ingredients:
- 1 ½ oz. can chicken breast
- 4 slices bacon
- ¼ cup parmesan cheese
- 1 large egg
- 3 tbsp flour

Directions:
1. Cook the bacon until crispy.
2. Chop the chicken and bacon together in a food processor until fine.
3. Add in the parmesan, egg, and flour, and mix.
4. Make the patties by hand and fry on medium heat in a skillet with some oil.
5. Once browned, flip over, continue cooking, and let them drain.
6. Serve!

Nutrition:
- Calories: 387
- Fat: 16 g
- Carbs: 13 g
- Protein: 34 g

321. Cheddar Bacon Burst

Difficulty: Easy
Preparation Time: 25 minutes
Cooking Time: 40 minutes
Servings: 8
Ingredients:
- 30 slices bacon
- 2 ½ cups cheddar cheese
- 4–5 cups raw spinach
- 1–2 tbsp Tone's Southwest Chipotle Seasoning
- 2 tsp Mrs. Dash Table Seasoning

Directions:
1. Preheat the fryer to 375°F/190°C.
2. Weave the bacon into 15 vertical pieces & 12 horizontal pieces. Cut the extra 3 in half to fill in the rest, horizontally.
3. Season the bacon.
4. Add the cheese to the bacon.
5. Add the spinach and press down to compress.
6. Tightly roll up the woven bacon.
7. Line a baking sheet with kitchen foil and add plenty of salt to it.
8. Put the bacon on top of a cooling rack and put that on top of your baking sheet.
9. Bake for 30–40 minutes.
10. Let cool for 10–15 minutes before
11. Slice and enjoy!

Nutrition:
- Calories: 218
- Fat: 9 g
- Carbs: 20 g
- Protein: 21 g

322. Quinoa with Vegetables

Difficulty: Medium
Preparation Time: 10 minutes
Cooking Time: 5 to 6 hours
Servings: 8
Ingredients:
- 2 cups quinoa, rinsed and drained
- 2 onions, chopped
- 2 carrots, peeled and sliced
- 1 cup sliced cremini mushrooms
- 3 garlic cloves, minced
- 4 cups low-sodium vegetable broth
- 1/2 tsp salt
- 1 tsp dried marjoram leaves
- 1/8 tsp freshly ground black pepper

Directions:
1. In a 6-quart slow cooker, mix all of the ingredients.
2. Cover and cook on low for 5 to 6 hours, or until the quinoa and vegetables are tender.
3. Stir the mixture and serve.

Nutrition:
- Calories: 204
- Carbohydrates: 35 g
- Sugar: 4 g
- Fiber: 4 g
- Fat: 3 g
- Saturated Fat: 0 g
- Protein: 7 g
- Sodium: 229 mg

323. Chicken Goulash

Difficulty: Easy
Preparation Time: 10 minutes
Cooking Time: 17 minutes
Servings: 6
Ingredients:
- 4 oz. chive stems
- 2 green peppers, chopped
- 1 tsp olive oil
- 14 oz. ground chicken
- 2 tomatoes
- ½ cup chicken stock
- 2 garlic cloves, sliced
- 1 tsp salt
- 1 tsp ground black pepper
- 1 tsp mustard

Directions:
1. Chop chives roughly.
2. Spray the air fryer basket tray with olive oil.
3. Preheat the air fryer to 365°F.
4. Put the chopped chives in the air fryer basket tray.
5. Add the chopped green pepper and cook the vegetables for 5 minutes.
6. Add the ground chicken.
7. Chop the tomatoes into small cubes and add them into the air fryer mixture too.
8. Cook the mixture for 6 minutes more.
9. Add the chicken stock, sliced garlic cloves, salt, ground black pepper, and mustard.
10. Mix well to combine.
11. Cook the goulash for 6 minutes more.

Nutrition:
- Calories: 161
- Fat: 6.1 g
- Carbs: 6 g
- Protein: 20.3 g

324. Chicken & Turkey Meatloaf

Difficulty: Easy
Preparation Time: 15 minutes
Cooking Time: 25 minutes
Servings: 12
Ingredients:
- 3 tbsp butter
- 10 oz. ground turkey
- 7 oz. ground chicken
- 1 tsp dried dill
- ½ tsp ground coriander
- 2 tbsp almond flour
- 1 tbsp minced garlic
- 3 oz. fresh spinach
- 1 tsp salt
- 1 egg
- ½ tbsp paprika
- 1 tsp sesame oil

Directions:
1. Put the ground turkey and ground chicken in a large bowl.
2. Sprinkle the meat with dried dill, ground coriander, almond flour, minced garlic, salt, and paprika.

3. Then chop the fresh spinach and add it to the ground poultry mixture.
4. Break the egg into the meat mixture and mix well until you get a smooth texture.
5. Great the air fryer basket tray with the olive oil.
6. Preheat the air fryer to 350°F.
7. Roll the ground meat mixture gently to make a flat layer.
8. Put the butter in the center of the meat layer.
9. Make the shape of the meatloaf from the ground meat mixture. Use your fingertips for this step.
10. Place the meatloaf in the air fryer basket tray.
11. Cook for 25 minutes.
12. When the meatloaf is cooked, allow it to rest before serving.

Nutrition:
- Calories: 142
- Fat: 9.8 g
- Carbs: 1.7 g
- Protein: 13 g

DESSERT RECIPES

325. Mint chocolate pudding cookies

Difficulty: Easy
Preparation Time: 10 minutes
Cooking Time: 10 minutes
Servings: 3 dozen
Ingredients:
- 1 cup sugar
- 1/2 cup butter—softened
- 1 egg
- 1/2 cup sour cream
- 3.4-ounce instant vanilla pudding mix
- 1/2 tsp salts
- 1/2 tsp baking soda
- 2 cups all-purpose flour
- 2 tsp mint extract
- 2 drops of blue coloring and 10–15 drops green coloring
- 1 1/2 cups chocolate chips

Directions:
1. First, cream the butter and sugar.
2. Add pudding mix, sour cream, and egg.
3. Mix the baking soda, salt, and flour into the bowl.
4. Add flour mixture into pudding mixture and combine well.
5. Add food coloring and mint extract.
6. Add in chocolate chips and add drops onto the greased cookie sheet.
7. Place in the oven and bake for ten minutes at 375°F.
8. Let cool it and serve!

Variation tip:
9. You don't add green drops coloring—skip it.
10. Serving Suggestion:
11. Serve with chia.

Nutrition:
- Calories 156
- Fat: 8 g
- Sodium: 110 mg
- Carbohydrates: 19 g
- Fiber: 1 g
- Sugar: 12 g
- Protein: 2 g

326. Tasty Pecan Pie Muffins

Difficulty: Easy
Preparation Time: 15 minutes
Cooking Time: 25 minutes
Servings: 9
Ingredients:
- 1 cup light brown sugar
- 1/2 cup all-purpose flour
- 1 cup pecan—chopped
- 2/3 cup butter—softened
- 2 eggs—beaten

Directions:
1. Preheat the oven to 350°F.
2. Grease and flour the eighteen mini muffin cups.
3. Add pecans, sugar, and flour into the bowl.
4. Next, beat the eggs and butter in another bowl. Add into dry ingredients and combine well.
5. Add the batter to prepared muffin cups.
6. Place into the oven and bake for twenty to twenty-five minutes at 350°F.

Variation Tip:
7. You can add almonds.

Serving Suggestion:
8. Sprinkle it with cinnamon sugar and whipped cream.

Nutrition:
- Calories 338
- Fat: 23.5 g
- Sodium: 119.3 mg
- Carbohydrates: 31.1 g
- Fiber: 1.4 g
- Sugar: 24.3 g
- Protein: 3.4 g

327. Yummy Lime Pie

Difficulty: Medium
Preparation Time: 10 minutes
Cooking Time: 5 hours
Servings: 8
Ingredients:
- 2 cups graham cracker crumbs
- 1/2 cup granulated sugar
- 1/2 cup salted butter—melted
- 14-ounce sweetened condensed milk
- 1/2 cup key lime juice
- 1 tbsp lime zest
- 8-ounce frozen whipped topping—divided
- 1 lime—sliced

Directions:
1. Preheat the oven to 325°F.
2. Add butter, sugar, and graham crackers crumb into the bowl and mix well.
3. Press the crumb mixture into the greased pie.
4. Place into the oven and bake for eighteen to twenty minutes.
5. Remove from the oven and cool it for a half hour.
6. Add lime zest, lime juice, and milk into the bowl and combine well.
7. Next, fold in two cups of whipped topping.
8. Transfer the mixture to pie crust and let cool for four hours.
9. Next, fill a piping bag with the remaining one cup of whipped cream and then top with lime slices.

Variation tip:
10. You can use fresh lime juice in this recipe.

Serving Suggestion:
11. Sprinkle it with lime zest.

Nutrition:
- Calories 481
- Fat: 24 g
- Sodium: 183 mg
- Carbohydrates: 60 g
- Fiber: 0 g
- Sugar 54 g
- Protein: 10 g

328. Fresh Green Grape Salad

Difficulty: Easy
Preparation Time: 15 minutes
Cooking Time: 0 minutes
Servings: 8
Ingredients:
- 4 pounds seedless green grapes
- 8-ounce cream cheese
- 8-ounce sour cream
- 1/2 cup white sugar
- 1 tsp vanilla extract
- 4 ounces pecans—chopped
- 2 tbsp brown sugar

Directions:
1. First, rinse and dry the grapes.
2. Combine the vanilla, sugar, sour cream, and cream cheese into the bowl.
3. Add grapes and combine well incorporated.
4. Sprinkle it with pecans and brown sugar and combine again.

Variation tip:
5. You can use red grapes too.

Serving Suggestion:
6. Sprinkle it with pecans and brown sugar.

Nutrition:
- Calories 481
- Fat: 24 g
- Sodium: 183 mg
- Carbohydrates: 60 g
- Fiber: 0 g
- Sugar: 54 g
- Protein: 10 g

329. Broccoli Cheese Waffles

Difficulty: Easy
Preparation Time: 5 minutes
Cooking Time: 5 minutes
Servings: 3 minutes
Ingredients:
- 1 cup broccoli—processed
- 1 cup cheddar cheese—shredded
- 1/3 cup parmesan cheese—grated
- 2 eggs—beaten

Directions:
1. First, spray the waffle iron with cooking spray. Preheat the waffle iron.

2. Add broccoli into the blender and blend until you reach the consistency of rice.
3. Combine all the ingredients into the bowl.
4. Add 1/3 of the mixture to the waffle iron and cook for four to five minutes until golden.

Serving Suggestions:
5. Sprinkle with ranch dressing or sour cream.

Nutrition:
- Calories 237
- Fat: 18 g
- Sodium: 211 mg
- Carbohydrates: 3 g
- Fiber: 1 g
- Sugar: 1 g
- Protein: 15 g

330. Hearty Fruit Salad

Difficulty: Easy
Preparation Time: 25 minutes
Cooking Time: 5 minutes
Additional Time: 3 hours
Servings: 10
Ingredients:
- 2/3 cup fresh orange juice
- 1/3 cup fresh lemon juice
- 1/3 cup packed brown sugar
- 1/2 tsp grated orange zest
- 1/2 tsp grated lemon zest
- 1 tsp vanilla extract
- 2 cups cubed fresh pineapple
- 2 cups strawberries—hulled and sliced
- 3 kiwi fruit—peeled and sliced
- 3 bananas—sliced
- 2 oranges—peeled and sectioned
- 1 cup seedless grape
- 2 cups blueberries

Directions:
1. Add lemon zest, orange, zest, brown sugar, lemon juice, and orange juice into the saucepan and boil over medium-high flame.
2. Decrease the speed of the flame to medium-low flame and simmer for five minutes.
3. Remove from the flame and add vanilla extract.
4. Keep it aside to cool.
5. Next, layer the fruit in the glass bowl—pineapple, blueberries, grapes, oranges, bananas, kiwi fruits, and strawberries.
6. Add sauce over the fruit and cover with a lid. Place into the refrigerator for three to four hours.

Variation tip:
7. You can use your favorite fruit.

Serving Suggestion:
8. Sprinkle it with pecans and crushed coconut.

Nutrition:
- Calories 155
- Fat: 0.6 g
- Sodium: 4.7 mg
- Carbohydrates: 39 g
- Fiber: 4.5 g
- Sugar: 28.7 g
- Protein 1.8 g

331. Vegan Waffles with Kale

Difficulty: Intermediate
Preparation Time: 5 minutes
Cooking Time: 10 minutes
Servings: 2
Ingredients:
For the Kale Mixture:
- 1.5 cups almond milk
- 1 cup kale—stems removed
- 1/2 tsp pink salt
- 3 drops vanilla essence
- 2 tsp apple cider vinegar
- 2 tbsp extra-virgin olive oil
- 1/4 cup fresh raspberries
- 1 tbsp brown sugar or coconut palm sugar

For the Batter:
- 1 1/4 cup all-purpose flour
- 2 tsp baking soda
- 1/4 cup almond milk

Directions:
1. Preheat the waffle iron.
2. Add all the ingredients for the kale mixture into the blender.
3. Blend on low speed until combined well.
4. Put a sieve over the glass bowl and then add all-purpose flour and baking powder. Sieve it.
5. When sieved, add kale mixture.
6. Whisk the batter until no lumps remain.

7. If the batter is thick, add the extra almond milk.
8. Brush the waffle iron with vegan butter.
9. Add batter to the waffle iron and cook for eight to ten minutes.
10. Serve!
11. Top with maple syrup and fresh fruits.
12. You can add applesauce, nutritional yeast, banana, chia seeds, hemp seeds, and flaxseed meal.

Variation tip:
13. You can add applesauce, nutritional yeast, banana, chia seeds, hemp seeds, and flaxseed meal.

Serving Suggestion:
14. Top with maple syrup and fresh fruits.

Nutrition:
- Calories 487
- Fat: 17 g
- Sodium: 2140 mg
- Carbohydrates: 71 g
- Fiber: 3 g
- Sugar: 6 g
- Protein: 10 g

332. **Best Chia Pudding**

Difficulty: Easy
Preparation Time: 10 minutes
Cooking Time: 0 minutes
Servings: 1
Ingredients:
- 3–4 tbsp chia seeds
- 1 cup milk
- 1/2 tbsp maple syrup or honey
- 1/4 tsp vanilla
- Toppings of choice: fresh berries or other fruit, granola, nut butter, etc.

Directions:
1. Add vanilla, maple syrup, milk, and chia seeds into the bowl or Mason jar.
2. Place the lid and shake the mixture well.
3. When mixed, let rest for five minutes.
4. Shake well and cover with a lid. Place the mixture into the refrigerator for one to two hours.
5. Add more chia seeds and stir well and place into the refrigerator for a half-hour.
6. Top with berries.
7. Place into the air-tight container and put into the refrigerator for five to seven days.

Variation tip:
8. You can use any kind of milk.

Serving Suggestion:
9. Top with fresh fruits.

Nutrition:
- Calories 271
- Fat: 16 g
- Sodium: 248 mg
- Carbohydrates: 26 g
- Fiber: 16 g
- Sugar: 6 g
- Protein: 10 g

333. **Sweet Potato Muffins**

Difficulty: Medium
Preparation Time: 10 minutes
Cooking Time: 25 minutes
Servings: 12
Ingredients:
- 2 ½ cups sweet potatoes—cooked and mashed
- ¾ cup coconut milk
- 1/2 tsp vanilla extract
- 1 ½ cups whole wheat flour
- 1/2 cup coconut sugar
- 1 tbsp baking powder
- 1 tsp ground cinnamon
- 1 pinch salt
- Almond butter—for topping

Directions:
1. Preheat the oven to 350°F and then add muffin liners to the muffin tin.
2. Add cooked mashed sweet potatoes with vanilla extract and coconut milk to the blender and blend until smooth.
3. Mix the salt, cinnamon, baking powder, sugar, and flour into the bowl.
4. Transfer the sweet potato mixture to the bowl of dry ingredients.
5. Stir well with a wooden spoon. Combine well.
6. Add batter into the muffin on tins-lined parchment paper.
7. Add one tsp of almond butter to the muffin.

8. Place into the oven and bake for twenty-five to thirty minutes.
9. Let cool them for fifteen to twenty minutes.

Variation tip:
10. For good results:
11. You can use yam potatoes instead of sweet potatoes.
12. You can add plant-based milk instead of coconut milk.
13. You can add coconut sugar.

Serving Suggestion:
14. Serve with your favorite topping.

Nutrition:
- Calories 126
- Fat: 3 g
- Sodium: 34 mg
- Carbohydrates: 23 g
- Fiber: 2 g
- Sugar: 5 g
- Protein: 2 g

334. **Gingerbread Biscotti**

Difficulty: Easy
Preparation Time: 25 minutes
Cooking Time: 40 minutes
Servings: 48
Ingredients:
- 1/3 cup vegetable oil
- 1 cup white sugar
- 3 eggs
- ¼ cup molasses
- 2 ¼ cups all-purpose flour
- 1 cup whole wheat flour
- 1 tbsp baking powder
- 1 ½ tbsp ground ginger
- ¾ tbsp ground cinnamon
- 1/2 tbsp ground cloves
- ¼ tsp ground nutmeg

Directions:
1. Preheat the oven to 375°F. Next, grease the cookie sheet.
2. Combine the molasses, eggs, sugar, and oil into the bowl.
3. Mix the nutmeg, cloves, cinnamon, ginger, baking powder, and flour in another bowl.
4. Combine into the egg mixture to make a stiff dough.
5. Split half dough and shape half into the cookie.
6. Put rolls on the cookie sheet and press down to flatten the dough to half-inch thickness. Place into the oven.
7. Bake for twenty minutes. When done, remove it from the oven and keep it aside.
8. When cooled, slice into half-inch thick.
9. Place on the cookie sheet and bake for five to seven minutes per side.

Variation tip:
10. Add chocolate dip if you prefer.

Serving Suggestion:
11. Serve with coffee.

Nutrition:
- Calories 70
- Fat: 2 g
- Sodium: 26.5 mg
- Carbohydrates: 12.1 g
- Fiber: 0.6 g
- Sugar: 5.2 g
- Protein: 1.4 g

335. **Sweet Pumpkin Waffles**

Difficulty: Easy
Preparation Time: 30 minutes
Cooking Time: 15 minutes
Servings: 6
Ingredients:
- 2 ½ cups all-purpose flour
- 4 tsp baking powder
- 2 tsp ground cinnamon
- 1 tsp ground allspice
- 1 tsp ground ginger
- 1/2 tsp salts
- ¼ cup brown sugar
- 1 cup pumpkin
- 2 cups milk
- 4 eggs—separated
- ¼ cup butter—melted

Apple cider syrup:
- 1/2 cup white sugar
- 1 tbsp cornstarch
- 1 tsp ground cinnamon
- 1 cup apple cider
- 1 tbsp lemon juice
- 2 tbsp butter

Directions:
1. Preheat the waffle iron.
2. Mix the brown sugar, salt, ginger, all-spice, cinnamon, baking powder, and flour into the mixing bowl.
3. Add egg yolks, milk, and pumpkin to another bowl.
4. Whip the egg whites in the bowl.
5. Add ¼ cup melted butter and flour mixture to the pumpkin mixture and combine well.
6. Add ⅓ of egg whites into the batter using a rubber spatula.
7. Add in the remaining egg whites and cook the waffles using a waffle iron.
8. For making syrup: Add cinnamon, cornstarch, and sugar into the sauce. Add lemon juice and apple cider and cook well until thick.
9. Remove from flame and then add two tbsp of butter and serve!

Variation tip:
10. You can add cloves instead of all-spice.

Serving Suggestion:
11. Serve with maple syrup or apple sauce.

Nutrition:
- Calories 530
- Fat: 17.1 g
- Sodium: 702.8 mg
- Carbohydrates: 82.3 g
- Fiber: 3.9 g
- Sugar: 36 g
- Protein: 13 g

336. Chia Pudding

Difficulty: Easy
Preparation Time: 20 minutes
Cooking Time: 0 minutes
Servings: 2
Ingredients:
- 4 tbsp chia seeds
- 1 cup unsweetened coconut milk
- 1/2 cup raspberries

Directions:
1. Add raspberry and coconut milk into a blender and blend until smooth.
2. Pour the mixture into the glass jar.
3. Add chia seeds to a jar and stir well.
4. Seal the jar with a lid, shake well and place in the refrigerator for 3 hours.
5. Serve chilled and enjoy.

Nutrition:
- Calories: 360
- Fat: 33 g
- Carbs: 13 g
- Sugar: 5 g
- Protein: 6 g
- Cholesterol: 0 mg

337. Avocado Pudding

Difficulty: Easy
Preparation Time: 20 minutes
Cooking Time: 0 minutes
Servings: 8
Ingredients:
- 2 ripe avocados, pitted and cut into pieces
- 1 tbsp fresh lime juice
- 14 oz. can coconut milk
- 2 tsp liquid stevia
- 2 tsp vanilla

Directions:
1. Inside the blender, add all the ingredients and blend until smooth.
2. Serve immediately and enjoy.

Nutrition:
- Calories: 317
- Fat: 30 g
- Carbs: 9 g
- Sugar: 0.5 g
- Protein: 3 g
- Cholesterol: 0 mg

338. Smooth Peanut Butter Cream

Difficulty: Easy
Preparation Time: 10 minutes
Cooking Time: 0 minutes
Servings: 8
Ingredients:
- 1/4 cup peanut butter
- 4 overripe bananas; chopped
- 1/3 cup cocoa powder
- 1/4 tsp vanilla extract
- 1/8 tsp salt

Directions:
1. Add all the listed ingredients to a blender and blend until smooth.
2. Serve immediately and enjoy.

Nutrition:
- Calories: 101
- Fat: 5 g
- Carbs: 14 g
- Sugar: 7 g
- Protein: 3 g
- Cholesterol: 0 mg

339. Raspberry Ice Cream

Difficulty: Easy
Preparation Time: 10 minutes
Cooking Time: 0 minutes
Servings: 2
Ingredients:
- 1 cup frozen raspberries
- 1/2 cup heavy cream
- 1/8 tsp stevia powder

Directions:
1. Blend all the listed ingredients in a blender until smooth.
2. Serve immediately and enjoy.

Nutrition:
- Calories: 144
- Fat: 11 g
- Carbs: 10 g
- Sugar: 4 g
- Protein: 2 g
- Cholesterol: 41 mg

340. Chocolate Frosty

Difficulty: Easy
Preparation Time: 20 minutes
Cooking Time: 0 minutes
Servings: 4
Ingredients:
- 2 tbsp unsweetened cocoa powder
- 1 cup heavy whipping cream
- 1 tbsp almond butter
- 5 drops liquid stevia
- 1 tsp vanilla

Directions:
1. Add cream into a medium bowl and beat using the hand mixer for 5 minutes.
2. Add the remaining ingredients and blend until a thick cream forms.
3. Pour in serving bowls and place them in the freezer for 30 minutes.
4. Serve and enjoy.

Nutrition:
- Calories: 137
- Fat: 13 g
- Carbs: 3 g
- Sugar: 0.5 g
- Protein: 2 g
- Cholesterol: 41 mg

341. Bounty Bars

Difficulty: Easy
Preparation Time: 20 minutes
Cooking Time: 0 minutes
Servings: 12
Ingredients:
- 1 cup coconut cream
- 3 cups shredded unsweetened coconut
- 1/4 cup extra virgin coconut oil
- 1/2 tsp vanilla powder
- 1/4 cup powdered erythritol
- 1 1/2 oz. cocoa butter
- 5 oz. dark chocolate

Directions:
1. Heat the oven to 350°F and toast the coconut in it for 5–6 minutes. Remove from the oven once toasted and put aside to cool.
2. Take a bowl of medium size and add coconut oil, coconut milk, vanilla, erythritol, and toasted coconut. Mix the ingredients well to form a smooth mixture.
3. With your hands, make 12 bars of equal size from the prepared mixture and adjust in the tray lined with parchment paper.
4. Place the tray in the fridge for about 1 hour and, in the meantime, put the cocoa butter and dark chocolate in a glass bowl.
5. Heat a cup of water in a saucepan over medium heat and place the bowl over it to melt the cocoa butter and dark chocolate.

6. Remove from the heat once melted properly, mix well until blended, and put aside to cool.
7. Take the coconut bars and coat them with dark chocolate mixture one by one using a wooden stick. Adjust on the tray lined with parchment paper and drizzle the remaining mixture over them.
8. Refrigerate for around 1 hour before you serve the delicious bounty bars.

Nutrition:
- Calories: 230
- Fat: 25 g
- Carbohydrates: 5 g
- Protein: 32 g

342. **Delicious Brownie Bites**

Difficulty: Easy
Preparation Time: 20 minutes
Cooking Time: 0 minutes
Servings: 13
Ingredients:
- 1/4 cup unsweetened chocolate chips
- 1/4 cup unsweetened cocoa powder
- 1 cup pecans; chopped
- 1/2 cup almond butter
- 1/2 tsp vanilla
- 1/4 cup monk fruit sweetener
- 1/8 tsp pink salt

Directions:
1. Add pecans, sweetener, vanilla, almond butter, cocoa powder, and salt into the food processor and process until well mixed.
2. Transfer the brownie mixture into the massive bowl. Add chocolate chips and fold well.
3. Make small-sized balls from the brownie mixture and place them onto a baking tray.
4. Place in the freezer for 20 minutes.
5. Serve and enjoy.

Nutrition:
- Calories: 108
- Fat: 9 g
- Carbs: 4 g
- Sugar: 1 g
- Protein: 2 g
- Cholesterol: 0 mg

343. **Chocolate Popsicle**

Difficulty: Medium
Preparation Time: 20 minutes
Cooking Time: 10 minutes
Servings: 6
Ingredients:
- 4 oz. unsweetened chocolate; chopped
- 6 drops liquid stevia
- 1 1/2 cups heavy cream

Directions:
1. Add cream into the microwave-safe bowl and microwave until it just starts to boil.
2. Add chocolate into the cream and put it aside for 5 minutes.
3. Add liquid stevia into the cream mixture and stir until chocolate is melted. Pour mixture into the Popsicle molds and place in the freezer for 4 hours or until set.
4. Serve and enjoy.

Nutrition:
- Calories: 198
- Fat: 21 g
- Carbs: 6 g
- Sugar: 0.2 g
- Protein: 3 g
- Cholesterol: 41 mg

344. **Pumpkin Balls**

Difficulty: Easy
Preparation Time: 15 minutes
Cooking Time: 0 minutes
Servings: 18
Ingredients:
- 1 cup almond butter
- 5 drops liquid stevia
- 2 tbsp coconut flour
- 2 tbsp pumpkin puree
- 1 tsp pumpkin pie spice

Directions:
1. Mix together the pumpkin puree and almond butter in a large bowl, until well mixed.
2. Add liquid stevia, pie spice, and coconut flour, and blend well.
3. Make small balls from the mixture and place them onto a baking tray.
4. Place in the freezer for 1 hour.

5. Serve and enjoy.

Nutrition:
- Calories: 96
- Fat: 8 g
- Carbs: 4 g
- Sugar: 1 g
- Protein: 2 g
- Cholesterol: 0 mg

345. Blueberry Muffins

Difficulty: Easy
Preparation Time: 15 minutes
Cooking Time: 35 minutes
Servings: 12
Ingredients:
- 2 eggs
- 1/2 cup fresh blueberries
- 1 cup heavy cream
- 2 cups almond flour
- 1/4 tsp lemon zest
- 1/2 tsp lemon extract
- 1 tsp baking powder
- 5 drops stevia
- 1/4 cup butter; melted

Directions:
1. Heat the cooker to 350°F. Line muffin tin with cupcake liners and put aside.
2. Add eggs into the bowl and whisk until well mixed.
3. Add the remaining ingredients and blend to mix.
4. Pour mixture into the prepared muffin tin and bake for 25 minutes.
5. Serve and enjoy.

Nutrition:
- Calories: 190
- Fat: 17 g
- Carbs: 5 g
- Sugar: 1 g
- Protein: 5 g
- Cholesterol: 55 mg

346. Vanilla Avocado Popsicles

Difficulty: Easy
Preparation Time: 20 minutes
Cooking Time: 0 minutes
Servings: 6
Ingredients:
- 2 avocados
- 1 tsp vanilla
- 1 cup almond milk
- 1 tsp liquid stevia
- 1/2 cup unsweetened cocoa powder

Directions:
1. Add all the listed ingredients to a blender and blend until smooth.
2. Pour the blended mixture into the Popsicle molds and place in the freezer until ready.
3. Serve and enjoy.

Nutrition:
- Calories: 130
- Fat: 12 g
- Carbs: 7 g
- Sugar: 1 g
- Protein: 3 g
- Cholesterol: 0 mg

347. Chocolate Almond Butter Brownie

Difficulty: Intermediate
Preparation Time: 10 minutes
Cooking Time: 16 minutes
Servings: 4
Ingredients:
- 1 cup bananas; overripe
- 1/2 cup almond butter; melted
- 1 scoop protein powder
- 2 tbsp unsweetened cocoa powder

Directions:
1. Preheat the air fryer to 325°F. Grease the air fryer baking pan and set it aside.
2. Blend all the ingredients in a blender until smooth.
3. Pour batter into the prepared pan and place in the air fryer basket and cook for 16 minutes.
4. Serve and enjoy.

Nutrition:
- Calories: 82
- Fat: 2 g
- Carbs: 11 g
- Sugar: 5 g
- Protein: 7 g
- Cholesterol: 16 mg

348. Peanut Butter Fudge

Difficulty: Easy
Preparation Time: 10 minutes
Cooking Time: 10 minutes
Servings: 20
Ingredients:
- 1/4 cup almonds; toasted and chopped
- 12 oz. smooth peanut butter
- 15 drops liquid stevia
- 3 tbsp coconut oil
- 4 tbsp coconut cream
- A pinch of salt

Directions:
1. Line the baking tray with parchment paper.
2. Melt coconut oil in a pan over low heat. Add peanut butter, coconut cream, liquid stevia, and salt to a saucepan. Stir well.
3. Pour the fudge mixture into the prepared baking tray and sprinkle chopped almonds on top.
4. Place the tray in the refrigerator for 1 hour or until ready to serve.
5. Slice and serve.

Nutrition:
- Calories: 131
- Fat: 12 g
- Carbs: 4 g
- Sugar: 2 g
- Protein: 5 g
- Cholesterol: 0 mg

349. Almond Butter Fudge

Difficulty: Easy
Preparation Time: 10 minutes
Cooking Time: 10 minutes
Servings: 18
Ingredients:
- 3/4 cup creamy almond butter
- 1 1/2 cups unsweetened chocolate chips

Directions:
1. Line an 8x4-inch pan with parchment paper and put it aside.
2. Add chocolate chips and almond butter into the double saucepan and cook over medium heat until the chocolate-butter mixture is melted. Stir well. Place mixture into the prepared pan and place in the freezer until ready to serve.
3. Slice and serve.

Nutrition:
- Calories: 197
- Fat: 16 g
- Carbs: 7 g
- Sugar: 1 g
- Protein: 4 g
- Cholesterol: 0 mg

350. Optavia Granola

Difficulty: Easy
Preparation Time: 5 minutes
Cooking Time: 8 minutes
Servings: 3
Ingredients:
- 1 package Medifast or Optavia Oatmeal
- 1 packet stevia
- 1 tsp vanilla extract
- 1/2 tsp apple spice or pumpkin pie spice

Directions:
1. Preheat the oven to 400°F. In a bowl, mix all the ingredients and add enough water to make the granola stay together.
2. Drop the granola onto a baking pan lined with parchment paper.
3. Bake for 8 minutes, but make sure to give the granola a good shake halfway into the cooking time for even browning.

Nutrition:
- Calories: 209
- Protein: 5.8 g
- Carbohydrates: 42 g
- Fat: 3.2 g
- Sugar: 6.2 g

351. Peanut Butter Brownie

Difficulty: Easy
Preparation Time: 15 minutes.
Cooking Time: 1 minute.
Servings: 4
Ingredients:
- 3 tbsp peanut butter powder
- 3 tbsp water
- 6 packets Octavia double chocolate brownie fueling
- 1 cup water

Directions:
1. Mix peanut butter powder with water and chocolate brownie in a bowl.
2. Divide this batter on a baking sheet lined with parchment paper into small mounds.
3. Cover and freeze for 40 minutes.
4. Serve.

Serving Suggestion:
5. Serve the brownies with chocolate dip.

Variation Tip:
6. Dip the brownies in white chocolate syrup.

Nutrition:
- Calories 361
- Fat: 10 g
- Sodium: 218 mg
- Carbs: 56 g
- Fiber: 10 g
- Sugar: 30 g
- Protein: 14 g

352. Chocolate Cherry Cookie

Difficulty: Easy
Preparation Time: 15 minutes.
Cooking Time: 12 minutes.
Servings: 4
Ingredients:
- 1 Optavia dark chocolate covered cherry shake
- ½ tsp baking powder
- 2 tbsp water

Directions:
1. At 350°F, preheat your oven.
2. Mix cherry shake with water and baking powder in a bowl.
3. Divide this batter on a baking sheet, lined with parchment paper, into 8 small cookies.
4. Bake these cookies for 12 minutes in the preheated oven.
5. Serve.
6. Serving Suggestion: Serve the cookies with fresh berries on top.

Variation Tip:
7. Add cherry preserves at the center of the cookies.

Nutrition:
- Calories 118
- Fat: 20 g
- Sodium: 192 mg
- Carbs: 23.7 g
- Fiber: 0.9 g
- Sugar: 19 g
- Protein: 5.2 g

353. Stuffed pears with almonds

Difficulty: Easy
Preparation Time: 15 minutes.
Cooking Time: 25 minutes.
Servings: 6
Ingredients:
- Spices
- 4 pinches cinnamon
- 3 ounces flour
- 3 ounces granulated sugar
- 2 tbsp soup brown sugar
- 3 ounces almonds, powdered
- 1 ½ ounce frilled almond
- 1 ½ ounces hazelnut
- 3 ½ ounces butter
- 6 pears

Directions:
1. Mix butter with cinnamon, sugars, flour, almonds, and hazelnut in a food processor.
2. Core the pears and divide the nut mixture into these pears.
3. Place the stuffed pears on a baking sheet.
4. Bake these pears for 25 minutes in the oven at 300°F.
5. Serve once cooled.

Serving Suggestion:
6. Serve the pears with a scoop of vanilla cream on top.

Variation Tip:
7. Add chopped pecans to the filling as well.

Nutrition:
- Calories 248
- Fat: 16 g
- Sodium: 95 mg
- Carbs: 38.4 g
- Fiber: 0.3 g
- Sugar: 10 g
- Protein: 14.1 g

354. <u>**Peanut Butter Cups**</u>

Difficulty: Easy
Preparation Time: 15 minutes.
Cooking Time: 12 minutes.
Servings: 4
Ingredients:
- 1/4 cup creamy peanut butter
- 5 ounces chocolate
- Cacao Nibs, Sea Salt

Directions:
1. Melt chocolate with peanut butter in a bowl by heating it in the microwave.
2. Mix well and divide this mixture into 12 mini muffin cups.
3. Cover and refrigerate for 1 hour.
4. Serve.

Serving Suggestion:
5. Serve the cups with chocolate or apple sauce.

Variation Tip:
6. Dip the bites in white chocolate syrup.

Nutrition:
- Calories 117
- Fat: 12 g
- Sodium: 79 mg
- Carbs 24.8 g
- Fiber: 1.1 g
- Sugar: 18 g
- Protein: 5 g

355. <u>**Medifast Rolls**</u>

Difficulty: Medium
Preparation Time: 15 minutes.
Cooking Time: 35 minutes.
Servings: 4
Ingredients:
- 3 eggs, separated
- 3 tbsp cream cheese
- A pinch cream of tartar
- 1 packet Splenda

Directions:
1. At 350°F, preheat your oven.
2. Beat separated egg whites with cream of tartar in a bowl until fluffy.
3. Blend yolks with Splenda and cream cheese in a bowl until pale.
4. Fold in egg whites and mix gently.
5. Layer a baking sheet with parchment paper.
6. Divide the batter onto the baking sheet into cookie rounds.
7. Bake these rolls for 35 minutes in the oven at 350°F.
8. Serve once cooled.

Serving Suggestion:
9. Serve the rolls with creamy frosting on top.

Variation Tip:
10. Add chopped pecans or walnuts to the batter.

Nutrition:
- Calories: 195
- Fat: 3 g
- Sodium: 355 mg
- Carbs: 20 g
- Fiber: 1 g
- Sugar: 25 g
- Protein: 1g

356. <u>**Apple Crisp**</u>

Difficulty: Easy
Preparation Time: 15 minutes.
Cooking Time: 40 minutes.
Servings: 4
Ingredients:
- 4 cups apples, peeled and sliced
- 1 tbsp coconut oil, melted
- 1/2 tsp cinnamon

- 1/4 tsp ground ginger

Crisp Topping
- ½ tsp cinnamon
- ¼ tsp ginger
- ¼ tsp nutmeg
- 1 cup old fashioned oats
- 1/3 cup pecans chopped
- 2 tbsp coconut oil
- 1 tbsp maple syrup

Directions:
1. At 350°F, preheat your oven. Grease an 8x8 inch baking dish.
2. Toss apples with coconut oil, ginger, and cinnamon in a bowl.
3. Spread the apples in the baking dish.
4. Mix all the crisp topping in a bowl and drizzle over the apples.
5. Cover this baking dish with aluminum foil and bake for 20 minutes at 350°F.
6. Uncover the hot dish and bake for another 20 minutes.
7. Serve.

Serving Suggestion:
8. Serve the apple crisp with chopped nuts on top.

Variation Tip:
9. Add dried raisins to the apple crisp.

Nutrition:
- Calories 203
- Fat: 8.9 g
- Sodium: 340 mg
- Carbs 24.7 g
- Fiber: 1.2 g
- Sugar: 11.3 g
- Protein: 5.3 g

357. Cherry Dessert

Difficulty: Easy
Preparation Time: 15 minutes.
Cooking Time: 0 minutes.
Servings: 4
Ingredients:
- 2 cups lite whipped topping, thawed
- 1 (8-ounce) package cream cheese, softened
- 1 package sugar-free cherry gelatin
- 1/2 cup boiling water

Directions:
1. Beat cream with cream cheese in a bowl until smooth.
2. Mix gelatin mix with boiling water in a bowl.
3. Add this prepared gelatin mixture to the cream cheese mixture.
4. Mix well and spread this mixture into a pie pan.
5. Cover and refrigerate the cream cheese for 2 hours.
6. Serve.

Serving Suggestion:
7. Serve the cherry dessert with fresh berries on top.

Variation Tip:
8. Add vanilla extracts to the dessert.

Nutrition:
- Calories: 153
- Fat: 1 g
- Sodium: 8 mg
- Carbs: 66 g
- Fiber: 0.8 g
- Sugar: 56 g
- Protein: 1 g

358. Vanilla Pudding

Difficulty: Easy
Preparation Time: 15 minutes.
Cooking Time: 8 minutes.
Servings: 4
Ingredients:
- 2 cups milk
- 1/4 tsp salt
- 1/2 cup milk
- 3 tbsp cornstarch
- 3/4 tsp pure vanilla extract
- 1/8 tsp stevia
- 2 tsp buttery spread

Directions:
1. Warm 2 cups of milk in a saucepan.
2. Mix cornstarch with ½ cup milk in a bowl and pour into the saucepan.
3. Cook this milk mixture for 3 minutes until it thickens,
4. Stir in the remaining ingredients, then mix well.
5. Allow this pudding to cool and serve.

Serving Suggestion:
6. Serve the pudding with chocolate syrup or berries on top.

Variation Tip:
7. Add crushed walnuts or pecans to the custard.

Nutrition:
- Calories: 198
- Fat: 14 g
- Sodium: 272 mg
- Carbs: 34 g
- Fiber: 1 g
- Sugar: 9.3 g
- Protein: 1.3 g

SNACK RECIPES

359. Sausage and Cheese Dip

Difficulty: Medium
Preparation Time: 10 minutes
Cooking Time: 130 minutes
Servings: 28
Ingredients:
- 8 ounces cream cheese
- A pinch of salt and black pepper
- 16 ounces sour cream
- 8 ounces pepper jack cheese; chopped
- 15 ounces canned tomatoes mixed with habaneros
- 1-pound Italian sausage; ground
- ¼ cup green onions; chopped

Directions:
1. Heat up a pan over medium heat, add sausage, stir and cook until it browns.
2. Add tomatoes, mix, stir and cook for 4 minutes more.
3. Add a pinch of salt, black pepper, and green onions, stir and cook for 4 minutes.
4. Spread pepper jack cheese on the bottom of your slow cooker.
5. Add cream cheese, sausage mix, and sour cream, cover, and cook on High for 2 hours.
6. Uncover your slow cooker, stir dip, transfer to a bowl, and serve.
7. Enjoy!

Nutrition:
- Calories: 132
- Protein: 6.79 g
- Fat: 9.58 g
- Carbohydrates: 6.22 g
- Sodium: 362 mg

360. Stuffed Avocado

Difficulty: Easy
Preparation Time: 10 minutes
Cooking Time: 0 minutes
Servings: 2
Ingredients:
- 1 avocado; halved and pitted
- 10 ounces canned tuna; drained
- 2 tbsp sun-dried tomatoes; chopped
- 1 ½ tbsp basil pesto
- 2 tbsp black olives; pitted and chopped
- Salt and black pepper to the taste
- 2 tsp pine nuts; toasted and chopped
- 1 tbsp basil; chopped

Directions:
1. In a bowl, mix the tuna with the sun-dried tomatoes and the rest of the ingredients except the avocado and stir.
2. Stuff the avocado halves with the tuna mix and serve as an appetizer.

Nutrition:
- Calories: 233
- Fat: 9 g
- Fiber: 3.5 g
- Carbs: 11.4 g
- Protein: 5.6 g

361. Tasty Onion and Cauliflower Dip

Difficulty: Easy
Preparation Time: 20 minutes
Cooking Time: 30 minutes
Servings: 24
Ingredients:
- 1 ½ cups chicken stock
- 1 cauliflower head; florets separated
- ¼ cup mayonnaise
- ½ cup yellow onion; chopped
- ¾ cup cream cheese
- ½ tsp chili powder
- ½ tsp cumin; ground
- ½ tsp garlic powder
- Salt and black pepper to the taste

Directions:
1. Put the stock in a pot, add cauliflower and onion, heat up over medium heat, and cook for 30 minutes.
2. Add chili powder, salt, pepper, cumin, and garlic powder, and stir.
3. Also, add cheese and stir a touch until it melts.

4. Blend using an immersion blender and blend with the mayo.
5. Transfer to a bowl and keep in the fridge for 2 hours before you serve it.
6. Enjoy!

Nutrition:
- Calories: 40
- Protein: 1.23 g
- Fat: 3.31 g
- Carbohydrates: 1.66 g
- Sodium: 72 mg

362. <u>Avocado Taco Boat</u>

Difficulty: Easy
Preparation Time: 5 minutes
Cooking Time: 20 minutes
Servings: 4
Ingredients:
- 4 grape tomatoes
- 2 large avocados
- 1 lb. ground beef
- 4 tbsp taco seasoning
- 3/4 cup shredded sharp cheddar cheese
- 4 slices pickled jalapeño
- 1/4 cup salsa
- 3 shredded romaine leaves
- 1/4 cup sour cream
- 2/3 cup water

Directions:
1. Take a skillet of huge size, grease it with oil, and warm it over medium-high heat. Cook the bottom beef in it for 10–15 minutes or until it has a brownish look.
2. Once the meat browns, drain the grease from the skillet and add the water and the taco seasoning.
3. Reduce the heat once the taco seasoning gets mixed well and simmer for 8–10 minutes.
4. Take both avocados and cut them in halves using a sharp knife.
5. Take each avocado shell and fill it with ¼ of the shredded romaine leaves.
6. Fill each shell with ¼ of the cooked ground beef.
7. Do the topping with soured cream, cheese, jalapeno, salsa, and tomato before you serve the delicious avocado taco.

Nutrition:
- Calories: 430
- Fat: 35 g
- Carbohydrates: 5 g
- Protein: 32 g

363. <u>Pesto Crackers</u>

Difficulty: Easy
Preparation Time: 10 minutes
Cooking Time: 17 minutes
Servings: 6
Ingredients:
- ½ tsp baking powder
- Salt and black pepper to the taste
- 1 and ¼ cups almond flour
- ¼ tsp basil; dried
- 1 garlic clove; minced
- 2 tbsp basil pesto
- A pinch cayenne pepper
- 3 tbsp ghee

Directions:
1. In a bowl, mix salt, pepper, baking powder, and almond flour.
2. Add garlic, cayenne, and basil and stir.
3. Add pesto and whisk.
4. Also, add ghee and blend your dough with your finger.
5. Spread this dough on a lined baking sheet, then put it in the oven at 325°F and bake for 17 minutes.
6. Set aside to cool, then cut your crackers and serve them as a snack.
7. Enjoy!

Nutrition:
- Calories: 9
- Protein: 0.41 g
- Fat: 0.14 g
- Carbohydrates: 1.86 g
- Sodium: 2 mg

364. Chicken and Mushrooms

Difficulty: Easy
Preparation Time: 10 minutes
Cooking Time: 15 minutes
Servings: 6
Ingredients:
- 2 chicken breasts
- 1 cup sliced white champignons
- 1 cup sliced green chilies
- 1/2 cup scallions; hacked
- 1 tsp chopped garlic
- 1 cup low-fat cheddar shredded cheese (1–1.5 lb. g Fat: / ounce)
- 1 tbsp olive oil
- 1 tbsp butter

Directions:
1. Fry the chicken breasts with olive oil.
2. Add salt and pepper as needed.
3. Grill breasts of chicken on a plate with a grill.
4. For every serving, weigh 4 ounces of chicken. (Make two servings, save leftovers for an additional meal).
5. In a buttered pan, stir in mushrooms, green peppers, scallions, and garlic until smooth, and a bit dark.
6. Place the chicken on a baking platter.
7. Cover with the mushroom combination.
8. Top with ham.
9. Place the cheese in a 350°F oven until it melts.

Nutrition:
- Carbohydrates: 2 g
- Protein: 23 g
- Fat: 11 g
- Cholesterol: 112 mg
- Sodium: 198 mg
- Potassium: 261 mg

365. Marinated Eggs

Difficulty: Easy
Preparation Time: 2 hours and 10 minutes
Cooking Time: 7 minutes
Servings: 4
Ingredients:
- 6 eggs
- 1 and ¼ cups water
- ¼ cup unsweetened rice vinegar
- 2 tbsp coconut aminos
- Salt and black pepper to the taste
- 2 garlic cloves; minced
- 1 tsp stevia
- 4 ounces cream cheese
- 1 tbsp chives; chopped

Directions:
1. Put the eggs in a pot, add water to cover, bring to a boil over medium heat, and cover and cook for 7 minutes.
2. Rinse eggs with cold water and set them aside to chill down.
3. In a bowl, mix one cup of water with coconut aminos, vinegar, stevia, and garlic, and whisk well.
4. Put the eggs in this mix, cover with a kitchen towel, and put them aside for 2 hours, turning from time to time.
5. Peel eggs, cut them in halves, and put egg yolks in a bowl.
6. Add ¼ cup water, cream cheese, salt, pepper, and chives, and stir well.
7. Stuff egg whites with this mix and serve them.
8. Enjoy!

Nutrition:
- Calories: 289
- Protein: 15.86 g
- Fat: 22.62 g
- Carbohydrates: 4.52 g
- Sodium: 288 mg

366. Chili Mango and Watermelon Salsa

Difficulty: Intermediate
Preparation Time: 5 minutes
Cooking Time: 0 minutes
Servings: 12
Ingredients:
- 1 red tomato; chopped
- Salt and black pepper to the taste
- 1 cup watermelon; seedless, peeled and cubed
- 1 red onion; chopped
- 2 mangos; peeled and chopped
- 2 chili peppers; chopped

- ¼ cup cilantro; chopped
- 3 tbsp lime juice
- Pita chips for serving

Directions:
1. In a bowl, mix the tomato with the watermelon, the onion, and the rest of the ingredients except the pita chips, and toss well.
2. Divide the mix into small cups and serve with pita chips on the side.

Nutrition:
- Calories: 62
- Fat: 4 g
- Fiber: 1.3 g
- Carbs: 3.9 g
- Protein: 2.3 g

367. Pumpkin Muffins

Difficulty: Easy
Preparation Time: 10 minutes
Cooking Time: 15 minutes
Servings: 18
Ingredients:
- ¼ cup sunflower seed butter
- ¾ cup pumpkin puree
- 2 tbsp flaxseed meal
- ¼ cup coconut flour
- ½ cup erythritol
- ½ tsp nutmeg; ground
- 1 tsp cinnamon; ground
- ½ tsp baking soda
- 1 egg ½ tsp baking powder
- A pinch of salt

Directions:
1. In a bowl, mix butter with pumpkin puree and egg and blend well.
2. Add flaxseed meal, coconut flour, erythritol, baking soda, baking powder, nutmeg, cinnamon, a pinch of salt, and stir well.
3. Spoon this into a greased muffin pan, put in the oven at 350°F, and bake for 15 minutes.
4. Leave muffins to chill down and serve them as a snack.
5. Enjoy!

Nutrition:
- Calories: 65
- Protein: 2.82 g
- Fat: 5.42 g
- Carbohydrates: 2.27 g
- Sodium: 57 mg

368. Chicken Enchilada Bake

Difficulty: Medium
Preparation Time: 20 minutes
Cooking Time: 50 minutes
Servings: 5
Ingredients:
- 5 oz. Shredded chicken breast (boil and shred ahead) or 99 percent fat-free white chicken can be used in a pan.
- 1 can tomato paste
- 1 low sodium chicken broth can be fat-free
- 1/4 cup cheese with low-fat mozzarella
- 1 tbsp oil
- 1 tbsp salt
- Ground cumin, chili powder, garlic powder, oregano, and onion powder (all to taste)
- 1 to 2 zucchinis sliced vertically (similar to lasagna noodles) into thin lines
- Sliced (optional) olives

Directions:
1. Add vegetable oil to a saucepan over medium-high heat, stir in ingredients and seasonings, and heat in chicken stock for 2–3 min.
2. Turn heat to low for 15 min, stirring regularly to boil.
3. Set aside and cool to ambient temperature.
4. Pull-strip of zucchini through enchilada sauce and lay flat on the pan's bottom in a small baking pan.
5. Next, add the chicken with 1/4 cup of enchilada sauce and blend it.
6. Place chicken on the end-to-end duvet of the baking tray.
7. Sprinkle some bacon over the chicken.
8. Add another layer of the pulled zucchini via enchilada sauce (similar to lasagna making).
9. When needed, cover with the remaining cheese and olives on top. Bake for 35 to 40 minutes.
10. Keep an eye on them.
11. When the cheese starts getting golden, cover with foil.

12. Serve and enjoy!

Nutrition:
- Calories: 312
- Carbohydrates: 21.3 g
- Protein: 27 g
- Fat: 10.2 g

369. Greek Tuna Salad Bites

Difficulty: Easy
Preparation Time: 5 Minutes
Cooking Time: 10 Minutes
Servings: 6
Ingredients:
- Cucumbers (2 medium)
- White tuna (2 to 6 oz. cans)
- Lemon juice (half of 1 lemon)
- Red bell pepper (.5 cup)
- Sweet/red onion (.25 cup)
- Black olives (.25 cup)
- Garlic (2 tbsp)
- Olive oil (2 tbsp)
- Fresh parsley (2 tbsp)
- Dried oregano
- salt & pepper (as desired)

Directions:
1. Drain and flake the tuna. Juice the lemon. Dice/chop the onions, olives, pepper, parsley, and garlic. Slice each of the cucumbers into thick rounds (skin off or on).
2. In a mixing container, mix the rest of the ingredients.
3. Place a heaping spoonful of salad onto the rounds and enjoy.

Nutrition:
- Calories: 400
- Fats: 22 g
- Carbs: 26 g
- Fiber Content: 8 g
- Protein: 30 g

370. Veggie Fritters

Difficulty: Easy
Preparation Time: 5 Minutes
Cooking Time: 10 minutes
Servings: 4
Ingredients:
- 2 garlic cloves; minced
- 2 yellow onions; chopped
- 4 scallions; chopped
- 2 carrots; grated
- 2 tsp cumin; ground
- ½ tsp turmeric powder
- Salt and black pepper to the taste
- ¼ tsp coriander; ground
- 2 tbsp parsley; chopped
- ¼ tsp lemon juice
- ½ cup almond flour
- 2 beets; peeled and grated
- 2 eggs; whisked
- ¼ cup tapioca flour
- 3 tbsp olive oil

Directions:
1. In a bowl, combine the garlic with the onions, scallions, and the rest of the ingredients except the oil. Stir well and shape medium fritters out of this mix.
2. Heat up a pan with the oil over medium-high heat, add the fritters, cook for 5 minutes on all sides, arrange on a platter and serve.

Nutrition:
- Calories: 209
- Fat: 11.2 g
- Fiber: 3 g
- Carbs: 4.4 g
- Protein: 4.8 g

371. Cucumber Sandwich Bites

Difficulty: Easy
Preparation Time: 5 minutes
Cooking Time: 0 minutes
Servings: 12
Ingredients:
- 1 cucumber; sliced
- 8 slices whole-wheat bread
- 2 tbsp cream cheese; soft
- 1 tbsp chives; chopped
- ¼ cup avocado; peeled, pitted and mashed
- 1 tsp mustard
- Salt and black pepper to the taste

Directions:
1. Spread the mashed avocado on each bread slice, also spread the rest of the ingredients except the cucumber slices.

2. Divide the cucumber slices into the bread slices, cut each slice in thirds, arrange on a platter and serve as an appetizer.

Nutrition:
- Calories: 187
- Fat: 12.4 g
- Fiber: 2.1 g
- Carbs: 4.5 g
- Protein 8.2 g

372. White Bean Dip

Difficulty: Easy
Preparation Time: 5 Minutes
Cooking Time: 0 minutes
Servings: 4
Ingredients:
- 15 ounces canned white beans; drained and rinsed
- 6 ounces canned artichoke hearts; drained and quartered
- 4 garlic cloves; minced
- 1 tbsp basil; chopped
- 2 tbsp olive oil
- Juice ½ lemon
- Zest ½ lemon; grated
- Salt and black pepper to the taste

Directions:
1. In your food processor, mix the beans with the artichokes and the rest of the ingredients except the oil and pulse well.
2. Add the oil gradually, pulse the combination again, divide into cups and serve with a celebration dip.

Nutrition:
- Calories: 274
- Fat: 11.7 g
- Fiber: 6.5 g
- Carbs: 18.5 g
- Protein: 16.5 g

373. Eggplant Dip

Difficulty: Easy
Preparation Time: 5 Minutes
Cooking Time: 40 minutes
Servings: 4
Ingredients:
- 1 eggplant; poked with a fork
- 2 tbsp tahini paste
- 2 tbsp lemon juice
- 2 garlic cloves; minced
- 1 tbsp olive oil
- Salt and black pepper to the taste
- 1 tbsp parsley; chopped

Directions:
1. Put the eggplant in a roasting pan, bake at 400°F for 40 minutes, allow to cool down, then peel and transfer to your food processor.
2. Add the rest of the ingredients except the parsley, pulse well, divide into small bowls and serve an appetizer with the parsley sprinkled on top.

Nutrition:
- Calories: 121
- Fat: 4.3 g
- Fiber: 1 g
- Carbs: 1.4 g
- Protein: 4.3 g

374. Feta Artichoke Dip

Difficulty: Easy
Preparation Time: 10 minutes
Cooking Time: 30 minutes
Servings: 8
Ingredients:
- 8 ounces artichoke hearts; drained and quartered
- ¾ cup basil; chopped
- ¾ cup green olives; pitted and chopped
- 1 cup parmesan cheese; grated
- 5 ounces feta cheese; crumbled

Directions:
1. In your food processor, mix the artichokes with the basil and the rest of the ingredients, pulse well, and transfer to a baking dish.
2. Put in the oven, bake at 375°F for 30 minutes, and serve as a party dip.

Nutrition:
- Calories: 186
- Fat: 12.4 g
- Fiber: 0.9 g
- Carbs: 2.6 g
- Protein: 1.5 g

375. Avocado Dip

Difficulty: Easy
Preparation Time: 5 minutes
Cooking Time: 0 minutes
Servings: 8
Ingredients:
- ½ cup heavy cream
- 1 green chili pepper; chopped
- Salt and pepper to the taste
- 4 avocados; pitted, peeled, and chopped
- 1 cup cilantro; chopped
- ¼ cup lime juice

Directions:
1. In a blender, mix the cream with the avocados and the rest of the ingredients, and pulse well.
2. Divide the mix into bowls and serve cold as a party dip.

Nutrition:
- Calories: 200
- Fat: 14.5 g
- Fiber: 3.8 g
- Carbs: 8.1 g
- Protein: 7.6 g

376. Green Beans Rice

Difficulty: Easy
Preparation Time: 10 minutes
Cooking Time: 20 minutes
Servings: 4
Ingredients:
- 4 cups water
- 2 cups green beans, trimmed and halved
- 2 cups brown rice
- 4 garlic cloves, minced
- 1 tsp nutmeg, ground
- Salt and black pepper to the taste

Directions:
1. In your instant pot, combine the rice with the rest of the ingredients except the green beans, shut the lid, and cook on High for 15 minutes
2. Release the pressure fast for 5 minutes, add the green beans, put the lid back on, and cook on High for 5 minutes more.
3. Release the pressure fast again for 5 minutes, divide the mix between plates and serve.

Nutrition:
- Calories: 190
- Fat: 6 g
- Carbs: 6 g
- Protein: 7 g

377. Garlic Kale

Difficulty: Easy
Preparation Time: 5 minutes
Cooking Time: 5 minutes
Servings: 4
Ingredients:
- 1-pound kale, roughly torn
- ¼ cup chicken stock
- 1 tbsp spring onion, chopped
- 4 garlic cloves, minced

Directions:
1. In your instant pot, combine all the ingredients, put the lid on, and cook on High for 5 minutes.
2. Release the pressure fast for 5 minutes, divide the mix between plates and serve.

Nutrition:
- Calories: 141
- Fat: 5 g
- Carbs: 6 g
- Protein: 6 g

378. Celery and Green Beans Mix

Difficulty: Easy
Preparation Time: 10 minutes
Cooking Time: 12 minutes
Servings: 4
Ingredients:
- 1-pound green beans, trimmed and halved
- 1 celery stalk, chopped
- 2 tbsp olive oil
- 1 red onion, chopped
- 1 cup chicken stock
- 1 tbsp rosemary, chopped
- Salt and black pepper to the taste

Directions:
1. Set the instant pot on cook mode, add the oil, heat it up, add the onion, stir and cook for 5 minutes.
2. Add the rest of the ingredients, put the lid on, and cook on High for 7 minutes
3. Release the pressure fast for 10 minutes, divide between plates and serve.

Nutrition:
- Calories: 162
- Fat: 4 g
- Carbs: 7 g
- Protein: 4 g

379. **Parmesan Asparagus**

Difficulty: Easy
Preparation Time: 5 minutes
Cooking Time: 8 minutes
Servings: 4
Ingredients:
- 3 garlic cloves, minced
- 1 bunch asparagus, trimmed
- 1 cup water
- 3 tbsp olive oil
- 3 tbsp parmesan, grated

Directions:
1. Put the water in your instant pot, add the steamer basket, add the asparagus inside, shut the lid and boil on High for 8 minutes.
2. Release the pressure fast for 5 minutes, transfer the asparagus to a container, add the rest of the ingredients, toss and serve as a side dish.

Nutrition:
- Calories: 13
- Fat: 4 g
- Carbs: 5 g
- Protein: 8 g

380. **Ginger Kale**

Difficulty: Medium
Preparation Time: 4 minutes
Cooking Time: 6 minutes
Servings: 4
Ingredients:
- 1-pound kale, torn
- ¼ cup veggie stock
- 2 tsp ginger, grated
- 2 garlic cloves, minced
- 1 tbsp balsamic vinegar
- Salt and white pepper to the taste

Directions:
1. In your instant pot, combine all the ingredients, put the lid on, and cook on High for 6 minutes.
2. Release the pressure fast for 4 minutes, divide the mix between plates and serve.

Nutrition:
- Calories: 120
- Fat: 4 g
- Carbs: 7 g
- Protein: 4 g

381. **Spicy Red Cabbage**

Difficulty: Easy
Preparation Time: 10 minutes
Cooking Time: 15 minutes
Servings: 4
Ingredients:
- 6 cups red cabbage, shredded
- ½ cup yellow onion, chopped
- 1 tbsp olive oil
- 1 tsp hot paprika
- Salt and black pepper to the taste
- 1 tbsp apple cider vinegar

Directions:
1. Set your instant pot in Stir-fry mode, add oil, heat, add onion, stir and sauté for 5 minutes
2. Add the remaining ingredients, stir, put the lid on and cook over high heat for 10 minutes. Leave the natural pressure for 10 minutes, divide the mixture between dishes and serve as a garnish.

Nutrition:
- Calories: 132
- Fat: 7 g
- Carbs: 6 g
- Protein: 8 g

APPETIZER RECIPES

382. Salmon Burger

Difficulty: Easy
Preparation Time: 15 minutes
Cooking Time: 15 minutes
Servings: 6
Ingredients:
- 16 ounces (450 g) pink salmon, minced
- 1 cup (250 g) prepared mashed potatoes
- 1 medium (110 g) onion, chopped
- 1 stalk celery (about 60 g), finely chopped
- 1 large egg (about 60 g), lightly beaten
- 2 tbsp (7 g) fresh cilantro, chopped
- 1 cup (100 g) breadcrumbs
- Vegetable oil, for deep frying
- Salt and freshly ground black pepper

Directions:
1. Combine the salmon, mashed potatoes, onion, celery, egg, and cilantro in a mixing bowl. Season to taste and mix thoroughly. Spoon about 2 tbsp mixture, roll in breadcrumbs, and then form into small patties.
2. Heat oil in a non-stick frying pan. Cook your salmon patties for 5 minutes on each side or until golden brown and crispy.
3. Serve in burger buns and with coleslaw on the side if desired.

Nutrition:
- Calories 230
- Fat: 7 g
- Carbs: 20 g
- Protein: 18 g

383. Salmon Sandwich with Avocado and Egg

Difficulty: Medium
Preparation Time: 15 minutes
Cooking Time: 10 minutes
Servings: 4
Ingredients:
- 8 ounces (250 g) smoked salmon, thinly sliced
- 1 medium (200 g) ripe avocado, thinly sliced
- 4 large poached eggs (about 60 g each)
- 4 slices whole-wheat bread (about 30 g each)
- 2 cups (60 g) arugula or baby rocket
- Salt and freshly ground black pepper

Directions:
1. Place 1 bread slice on a plate top with arugula, avocado, salmon, and poached egg. Season with salt and pepper. Repeat the procedure for the remaining ingredients.
2. Serve and enjoy.

Nutrition:
- Calories: 310
- Fat: 18 g
- Carbs: 7 g
- Protein: 12 g

384. Spinach and Cottage Cheese Sandwich

Difficulty: Intermediate
Preparation Time: 15 minutes
Cooking Time: 10 minutes
Servings: 4
Ingredients:
- 4 ounces (125 g) cottage cheese
- 1/4 cup (15 g) chives, chopped
- 1 tsp (5 g) capers
- 1/2 tsp (2.5 g) grated lemon rind
- 4 (2 oz. or 60 g) smoked salmon
- 2 cups (60 g) loose baby spinach
- 1 medium (110 g) red onion, sliced thinly
- 8 slices rye bread (about 30 g each)
- Kosher salt and freshly ground black pepper

Directions:
1. Preheat your griddle or Panini press.
2. Mix together cottage cheese, chives, capers, and lemon rind in a small bowl.
3. Spread and divide the cheese mixture into 4 bread slices. Top with spinach, onion slices, and smoked salmon.
4. Cover with the remaining bread slices.
5. Grill the sandwiches until golden and grill marks form on both sides.
6. Transfer to a serving dish.

7. Serve and enjoy.

Nutrition:
- Calories 386
- Fat: 1 g
- Carbs: 18 g
- Protein: 1 g

385. Feta and Pesto Wrap

Difficulty: Easy
Preparation Time: 15 minutes
Cooking Time: 10 minutes
Servings: 4
Ingredients:
- 8 ounces (250 g) smoked salmon filet, thinly sliced
- 1 cup (150 g) feta cheese
- 8 (15 g) Romaine lettuce leaves
- 4 (6-inch) pita bread
- 1/4 cup (60 g) basil pesto sauce

Directions:
1. Place 1 pita bread on a plate. Top with lettuce, salmon, feta cheese, and pesto sauce. Fold or roll to enclose filling. Repeat the procedure for the remaining ingredients.
2. Serve and enjoy.

Nutrition:
- Calories: 408
- Fat: 2 g
- Carbs: 1 g
- Protein: 11 g

386. Cheese and Onion on Bagel

Difficulty: Easy
Preparation Time: 15 minutes
Cooking Time: 10 minutes
Servings: 4
Ingredients:
- 8 ounces (250 g) smoked salmon filet, thinly sliced
- 1/2 cup (125 g) cream cheese
- 1 medium (110 g) onion, thinly sliced
- 4 bagels (about 80 g each), split
- 2 tbsp (7 g) fresh parsley, chopped
- Freshly ground black pepper to taste

Directions:
1. Spread the cream cheese on each bottom half of the bagel. Top with salmon and onion, season with pepper, sprinkle with parsley and then cover with bagel tops.
2. Serve and enjoy.

Nutrition:
- Calories: 34
- Carbs: 0 g
- Fat: 1 g
- Protein: 5 g

387. Bananas in Nut Cups

Difficulty: Easy
Preparation Time: 30 minutes
Cooking Time: 45 minutes
Servings: 6 servings
Ingredients:
- 3/4 cup shelled pistachios
- 1/2 cup sugar
- 1 tsp ground cinnamon
- 4 sheets phyllo dough, (14 inches x 9 inches)
- 1/4 cup butter, melted

Sauce:
- 3/4 cup butter, cubed
- 3/4 cup packed brown sugar
- 3 medium firm bananas, sliced
- 1/4 tsp ground cinnamon
- 3 to 4 cups vanilla ice cream

Directions:
1. Finely chop sugar and pistachios in a food processor; move to a bowl, then mix in cinnamon. Slice each phyllo sheet into 6 four-inch squares, and get rid of the trimmings. Pile the squares, then use plastic wrap to cover.
2. Pile 3 squares, and flip each at an angle to misalign the corners. Force each stack on the sides and bottom of an oiled eight-oz. custard cup. Bake for 15–20 minutes in a 350°F oven until golden; cool for 5 minutes. Move to a wire rack to cool completely.
3. Melt and boil brown sugar and butter in a saucepan to make the sauce at lower heat. Mix in cinnamon and bananas gently; heat completely. Put ice cream in the phyllo cups

until full, then put banana sauce on top. Serve right away.

Nutrition:
- Calories: 100
- Fat: 12 g
- Carbs: 2 g
- Protein: 4 g

388. Apple Salad Sandwich

Difficulty: Intermediate
Preparation Time: 15 minutes
Cooking Time: 10 minutes
Servings: 4
Ingredients:
- 4 ounces (125 g) canned pink salmon, drained and flaked
- 1 medium (180 g) red apple, cored and diced
- 1 celery stalk (about 60 g), chopped
- 1 shallot (about 40 g), finely chopped
- 1/3 cup (85 g) light mayonnaise
- 8 slices whole-grain bread (about 30 g each), toasted
- 8 (15 g) Romaine lettuce leaves
- Salt and freshly ground black pepper

Directions:
1. Combine the salmon, apple, celery, shallot, and mayonnaise in a mixing bowl. Season with salt and pepper.
2. Place 1 slice of bread on a plate, top with lettuce and salmon salad, and then cover with another slice of bread. Repeat the procedure for the remaining ingredients. Serve and enjoy.

Nutrition:
- Calories: 121
- Fat: 1 g
- Carbs: 18 g
- Protein: 1 g

389. Buttermilk Ice Cream Shake

Difficulty: Easy
Preparation Time: 5 minutes
Cooking Time: 0 minutes
Servings: 4
Ingredients:
- 3 cups chilled buttermilk
- 1/2 cup cold lemon juice
- A pinch salt
- 1/2 cup sugar
- 1/8 tsp grated lemon zest
- 1 cup vanilla ice cream
- Dash ginger

Directions:
1. Blend or shake all of the ingredients. Serve the shake together with the ginger.

Nutrition:
- Calories: 332
- Fat: 8 g
- Carbs: 1 g
- Protein: 14 g

390. Buttermilk Shake

Difficulty: Easy
Preparation Time: 5 minutes
Cooking Time: 0 minutes
Servings: 4
Ingredients:
- 1-pint vanilla ice cream
- 1 cup buttermilk
- 1 tsp grated lemon zest
- 1/2 tsp vanilla extract
- 1 drop lemon extract

Directions:
1. In a blender container, combine all the ingredients and process them at high speed until smooth. Pour the drink into the glasses. Make sure to put all the leftovers inside the refrigerator.

Nutrition:
- Calories: 309
- Fat: 26 g
- Carbs: 9 g
- Protein: 12 g

391. Cantaloupe Orange Milk Shakes

Difficulty: Easy
Preparation Time: 5 minutes
Cooking Time: 0 minutes
Servings: 4
Ingredients:
- 4 1/2 tsp orange juice concentrate
- 3/4 cup cubed cantaloupe
- 1 cup vanilla ice cream or frozen yogurt
- 3/4 cup milk
- 3 tbsp sugar

Directions:
1. Mix cantaloupe and orange juice concentrate in a blender. Cover the blender and process it until smooth. Add the sugar, milk, and ice cream. Cover again and process until well-blended. Pour the mixture into the chilled glasses and serve.

Nutrition:
- Calories: 252
- Fat: 9 g
- Carbs: 2 g
- Protein: 11 g

392. Cheese on Rye Bread

Difficulty: Easy
Preparation Time: 15 minutes
Cooking Time: 10 minutes
Servings: 4
Ingredients:
- 8 ounces (250 g) smoked salmon, thinly sliced
- 1/3 cup (85 g) mayonnaise
- 2 tbsp (30 ml) lemon juice
- 1 tbsp (15 g) Dijon mustard
- 1 tsp (3 g) garlic, minced
- 4 slices cheddar cheese (about 2 oz. or 30 g each)
- 8 slices rye bread (about 2 oz. or 30 g each)
- 8 (15 g) Romaine lettuce leaves
- Salt and freshly ground black pepper

Directions:
1. Mix together the mayonnaise, lemon juice, mustard, and garlic in a small bowl. Flavor with salt and pepper and set aside.
2. Spread dressing on 4 bread slices. Top with lettuce, salmon, and cheese. Cover with the remaining rye bread slices.
3. Serve and enjoy.

Nutrition:
- Calories: 321
- Fat: 1 g
- Carbs: 8 g
- Protein: 5 g

393. Buckwheat Granola

Difficulty: Easy
Preparation Time: 15 minutes
Cooking Time: 30 minutes
Servings: 10
Ingredients:
- 2 cups raw buckwheat groats
- ¾ cup pumpkin seeds
- ¾ cup almonds, chopped
- 1 cup unsweetened coconut flakes
- 1 tsp ground cinnamon
- 1 tsp ground ginger
- 1 ripe banana, peeled
- 2 tbsp maple syrup
- 2 tbsp olive oil

Directions:
1. Preheat your oven to 350°F. In a bowl, place the buckwheat groats, coconut flakes, pumpkin seeds, almonds, and spices, and mix well.
2. In another bowl, add the banana, and with a fork, mash well.
3. Add to the buckwheat mixture maple syrup and oil, and mix until well combined.
4. Transfer the mixture onto the prepared baking sheet and spread it in an even layer. Bake for about 25–30 minutes, stirring once halfway through.
5. Remove the baking sheet from the oven and set it aside to cool.

Nutrition:
- Calories: 342
- Fat: 7 g
- Carbs: 8 g
- Protein: 10 g

394. Apple Pancakes

Difficulty: Easy
Preparation Time: 15 minutes
Cooking Time: 24 minutes
Servings: 6
Ingredients:
- ½ cup buckwheat flour
- 2 tbsp coconut sugar
- 1 tsp baking powder
- ½ tsp ground cinnamon
- 1/3 cup unsweetened almond milk
- 1 egg, beaten lightly
- 2 granny smith apples, peeled, cored, and grated

Directions:
1. In a bowl, place the flour, coconut sugar, and cinnamon, and mix well.
2. In another bowl, place the almond milk and egg and beat until well combined.
3. Now, place the flour mixture and mix until well combined.
4. Fold in the grated apples.
5. Cook for 1–2 minutes on each side.
6. Repeat with the remaining mixture.
7. Serve warm with the drizzling of honey.

Nutrition:
- Calories: 588
- Fat: 3 g
- Carbs: 8 g
- Protein: 20 g

395. Matcha Pancakes

Difficulty: Easy
Preparation Time: 10 minutes
Cooking Time: 25 minutes
Servings: 6
Ingredients:
- 1 cup spelt flour
- 1 cup buckwheat flour
- 1 tbsp matcha powder
- 1 tbsp baking powder
- A pinch of salt
- ¾ cup unsweetened almond milk
- 1 tbsp olive oil
- 1/3 cup raw honey

Directions:
1. In a bowl, add the flax meal and warm water and mix well. Set aside for about 5 minutes.
2. Now, place the flour mixture and mix until a smooth textured mixture is formed.
3. Cook for about 2–3 minutes.
4. Carefully flip the side and cook for about 1 minute.
5. Repeat with the remaining mixture.
6. Serve warm with the drizzling of honey.

Nutrition:
- Calories: 345
- Fat: 12 g
- Carbs: 4 g
- Protein: 11 g

396. Smoked Salmon & Kale Scramble

Difficulty: Intermediate
Preparation Time: 10 minutes
Cooking Time: 9 minutes
Servings: 3
Ingredients:
- 2 cups fresh kale, tough ribs removed and chopped finely
- 1 tbsp coconut oil
- Ground black pepper to taste
- ½ cup smoked salmon, crumbled
- 4 eggs, beaten

Directions:
1. In a wok, melt the coconut oil over high heat and cook the kale with black pepper for about 3–4 minutes.
2. Stir in the smoked salmon and reduce the heat to medium.
3. Add the eggs and cook for about 3–4 minutes, stirring frequently.
4. Serve immediately.

Nutrition:
- Calories: 568
- Fat: 3 g
- Carbs: 5 g
- Protein: 10 g

397. Kale & Mushroom Frittata

Difficulty: Medium
Preparation Time: 15 minutes
Cooking Time: 30 minutes
Servings: 5
Ingredients:
- 8 eggs
- ½ cup unsweetened almond milk
- Salt and ground black pepper to taste
- 1 tbsp olive oil
- 1 onion, chopped
- 1 garlic clove, minced
- 1 cup fresh mushrooms, chopped
- 1½ cups fresh kale, tough ribs removed and chopped

Directions:
1. Preheat the oven to 350°F.
2. In a large bowl, place the eggs, coconut milk, salt, and black pepper, and beat well. Set aside.
3. In a large ovenproof wok, heat the oil over medium heat and sauté the onion and garlic for about 3–4 minutes.
4. Add the squash, kale, bell pepper, salt, and black pepper, and cook for about 8–10 minutes.
5. Stir in the mushrooms and cook for about 3–4 minutes.
6. Add the kale and cook for about 5 minutes.
7. Place the egg mixture on top evenly and cook for about 4 minutes, without stirring.
8. Transfer the wok to the oven and bake for about 12–15 minutes or until desired doneness.
9. Remove from the oven and place the frittata side for about 3–5 minutes before serving. Cut into desired-sized wedges and serve.

Nutrition:
- Calories: 356
- Fat: 2 g
- Carbs: 4 g
- Protein: 8 g

398. Kale, Apple, & Cranberry Salad

Difficulty: Easy
Preparation Time: 15 minutes
Cooking Time: 15 minutes
Servings: 4
Ingredients:
- 6 cups fresh baby kale
- 3 large apples, cored and sliced
- ¼ cup unsweetened dried cranberries
- ¼ cup almonds, sliced
- 2 tbsp extra-virgin olive oil
- 1 tbsp raw honey
- Salt and ground black pepper to taste

Directions:
1. In a salad bowl, place all the ingredients and toss to coat well.
2. Serve immediately.

Nutrition:
- Calories: 209
- Fat: 2 g
- Carbs: 5 g
- Protein: 8 g

399. Arugula, Strawberry, & Orange Salad

Difficulty: Intermediate
Preparation Time: 15 minutes
Cooking Time: 15 minutes
Servings: 4
Ingredients:
Salad:
- 6 cups fresh baby arugula
- 1½ cups fresh strawberries, hulled and sliced
- 2 oranges, peeled and segmented

Dressing:
- 2 tbsp fresh lemon juice
- 1 tbsp raw honey
- 2 tsp extra-virgin olive oil
- 1 tsp Dijon mustard
- Salt and ground black pepper to taste

Directions:
1. For the salad: In a salad bowl, place all the ingredients and mix.
2. For the dressing: place all the ingredients in another bowl and beat until well combined.

3. Place dressing on top of the salad and toss to coat well.
4. Serve immediately.

Nutrition:
- Calories: 389
- Fat: 8 g
- Carbs: 4 g
- Protein: 7 g

Nutrition:
- Calories: 84
- Protein: 13.4 g
- Carbs: 3.6 g
- Fat: 1.7 g
- Sugar: 0.8 g

400. <u>Lean and Green Crockpot Chili</u>

Difficulty: Easy
Preparation Time: 3 minutes
Cooking Time: 45 minutes
Servings: 8
Ingredients:
- 1-pound boneless skinless chicken breasts, cut into strips
- ½ cup chopped onion
- 2 tsp ground cumin
- 1 tsp minced garlic
- ½ tsp chili powder
- Salt and pepper to taste
- 1 ½ cups water
- 1 can green enchilada sauce
- ½ cup dried beans, soaked overnight

Directions:
1. Place all the ingredients in a pot.
2. Mix all the ingredients until combined.
3. Close the lid and turn on the heat to medium.
4. Bring to a boil and allow to simmer for 45 minutes or until the beans are cooked.
5. Serve with chopped cilantro on top.

SOUPS AND SALADS RECIPES

401. California Soup

Difficulty: Easy
Preparation Time: 10 min
Cooking Time: 10 min
Servings: 3
Ingredients:
- 1 quart (960 ml) chicken broth, heated
- 1 large or 2 small, very ripe black avocados, pitted, peeled, and cut into chunks

Directions:
1. Add the avocados with the broth in a blender puree until very smooth and serve.

Nutrition:
- Carbs: 3,5 g
- Fiber: 1,5 g
- Carbs: 2,5 g
- Protein: 4 g

402. Cheesy Cauliflower Soup

Difficulty: Medium
Preparation Time: 15 min
Cooking Time: 1 hour
Servings: 5
Ingredients:
- 1 tbsp (6 g) minced scallion
- 4 slices bacon, cooked and drained
- Guar or xanthan (optional)
- 1½ cups (180 g) shredded cheddar cheese
- 1½ cups (360 ml) Carb Countdown dairy beverage or half-and-half
- 1 tsp white vinegar
- 1 tsp salt
- 3 cups (720 ml) chicken broth
- 1 tbsp (7 g) grated carrot
- 2 tbsp (20 g) finely chopped celery
- 1 tbsp (10 g) finely chopped onion
- 600 g cauliflower, diced small

Directions:
1. In a big, heavy-bottomed pan, place the cauliflower, onion, celery, and carrot. Add the broth, salt, and vinegar to the chicken; bring it to a simmer and cook for about 30 to 45 minutes.
2. Stir in the Carb Countdown or half-and-half and then whisk in the cheese a bit at a time before adding more, allowing each additional time to melt. With guar or xanthan, thicken it a bit if you think it needs it.
3. Cover each serving with slightly crumbled bacon and hazelnuts.

Nutrition:
- Protein: 17 g
- Carbs: 7 g
- Fiber: 2 g

403. Egg drop Soup

Difficulty: Easy
Preparation Time: 10 min
Cooking Time: 10 min
Servings: 3
Ingredients:
- 3 Eggs
- 1 scallion, sliced
- ½ tsp grated fresh ginger
- 1 tbsp (15 ml) rice vinegar
- 1 tbsp (15 ml) soy sauce
- ¼ tsp guar (optional)
- 1 quart (960 ml) chicken broth

Directions:
1. Put 1 cup (240 ml) or so of the chicken stock in your processor, turn it on medium, and add the guar (if using). Let it mix for a moment, and then put it in a big saucepan with the broth's rest. (If you're not using the guar, then put all the liquid directly in a saucepan.)
2. Put in the rice vinegar, soy sauce, ginger, and scallion. Heat over medium-high heat and let it boil for 5–10 minutes to let the flavors mix.
3. Beat the eggs in a glass mixing cup or small pitcher—something with a pouring edge. Use a fork to stir the soup's surface in a gradual circle and pour in about ¼ of the eggs, stirring while cooking and turning them into shreds (which can occur almost instantly). Do three more times, using up half the egg.

Nutrition:
- Carbs: 2 g
- Protein: 8 g

404. Cauliflower, Spinach, and Cheese Soup

Difficulty: Intermediate
Preparation Time: 6 hours
Cooking Time: 1 1/2 hour
Servings: 8
Ingredients:
- 1 cup (240 ml) Carb Countdown dairy beverage
- 1 cup Gouda cheese
- 675 g shredded smoked
- 2 garlic cloves, crushed
- ¼ tsp pepper
- ½ tsp salt or Vega-Sal
- ¼ tsp cayenne
- 140 g bagged baby spinach leaves, pre-washed
- ½ cup (80 g) minced red onion
- 1 quart (960 ml) chicken broth
- Guar or xanthan
- 900 g cauliflower florets, cut into ½-inch (1.3-cm) pieces

Directions:
1. Combine the broth, cauliflower, onion, spinach, cayenne, or Vega-Sal salt, pepper, and garlic in your slow cooker. Close the slow cooker, set it to low, and let simmer for 6 hours or until tender.
2. Stir in the Gouda when the time's up, a little at a time, and then the Carb Timer. Cover the slow cooker again and steam for another 15 minutes or until the cheese has melted completely. Slightly thicken the broth with guar or xanthan.

Nutrition:
- Protein: 17 g
- Carbs: 7 g
- Fiber: 2 g
- Usable carbs: 5 g

405. Corner-Filling Soup

Difficulty: Easy
Preparation Time: 1/2 hour
Cooking Time: 1/2 hour
Servings: 6
Ingredients:
- ¼ tsp pepper
- 30 ml dry sherry
- 1 quart (960 ml) beef broth
- 1 small onion, sliced paper-thin
- 115 g sliced mushrooms
- 2 tbsp (28 g) butter

Directions:
1. In a pot, heat the butter and sauté the mushrooms and onions in the butter until they're soft.
2. Apply the broth, sherry, and pepper over the meat. For 5–10 minutes or so, let it steam, just to change the flavors a bit, and serve.

Nutrition:
- Carbs: 5,5 g
- Fiber: 1,1 g
- Usable carbs: 4,5 g
- Protein: 8 g

406. Stracciatella

Difficulty: Easy
Preparation Time: 15 min
Cooking Time: 45 min
Servings: 4–6
Ingredients:
- ½ tsp dried marjoram
- A pinch nutmeg
- ½ tsp lemon juice
- ½ cup (50 g) grated Parmesan cheese
- 2 Eggs
- 1 quart (960 ml) chicken broth, divided

Directions:
1. In a glass measuring cup or large pitcher, place 1/4 cup (60 ml) of the broth. Over medium heat, spill the remainder into a large saucepan.
2. In a measuring cup, add the eggs to the broth and beat them with a fork. Apply the lemon juice, Parmesan, and nutmeg, and then beat until well mixed using a fork.

3. Stir it using a fork as you add small quantities of the egg and cheese mixture until it is all mixed in while the broth in the saucepan is boiling. (Don't allow this to create long scraps like Chinese egg drop soup; instead, it makes small, fluffy particles because of the Parmesan.)
4. Apply the marjoram, smash it between your fingers a little bit, and steam the soup for a minute or two before serving.

Nutrition:
- Carbs: 2 g
- A trace of fiber
- Protein: 2 g

407. Peanut Soup

Difficulty: Easy
Preparation Time: 15 min
Cooking Time: 45 min
Servings: 5–7
Ingredients:
- Salted peanuts, chopped
- 420 ml half-and-half or heavy cream
- 1 tsp guar gum (optional)
- 1¼ cups (325 g) natural peanut butter (Here, we used it smoothly)
- ½ tsp salt or Vega-Sal
- 1.9 L chicken broth
- 1 medium onion, finely chopped
- 2 or 3 ribs celery, finely chopped
- 42 g butter

Directions:
1. Melt the butter in a pot, then sauté the butter with the celery and onion.
2. Stir in the broth, salt, and peanut butter.
3. Cover and cook for at least 60 minutes at the lowest temperature, stirring now and then.
4. If you are using guar gum (without adding carbohydrates, it makes the soup thicker; scoop 1 cup (245 ml) of the soup out of the pot about 16 minutes before serving.
5. To this cup, apply the guar gum, run the mixture for a couple of seconds through the blender and whisk it back into the broth.
6. Stir in half-and-a-half and cook for 15 minutes more. Connect the peanuts to the garnish.

Nutrition:
- Carbs: 19 g
- Fiber: 3 g
- Available Carbohydrates: 6 g
- Protein: 29 g

408. Soap De Frijoles Negros

Difficulty: Medium
Preparation Time: 15 min
Cooking Time: 45 min
Servings: 6–8
Ingredients:
- ¼ cup (16 g) chopped cilantro
- ½ cup (115 g) plain yogurt
- ½ tsp salt or Vega-Sal
- ½ tsp red pepper flakes
- 1 tbsp (6.3 g) ground cumin
- 30 ml lime juice
- 1 cup (130 g) salsa
- 2 Garlic cloves, crushed
- ½ cup (80 g) chopped onion
- 1 tbsp (15 ml) olive oil
- 1 can (14½ ounces, or 411 ml) chicken broth
- 1 can (15 ounces, or 420 g) black beans
- 2 cans (15 ounces, or 420 g) Eden brand black soybeans

Directions:
1. With the S-blade in place, bring half of the beans and half of the chicken broth into your blender or in your food processor. Run the unit before it purées the beans. Transfer the mixture and purée the other half of the beans and the other half of the chicken broth into a bowl that contains at least 2 quarts (1.9 L). To the first batch, add it.
2. Heat the olive oil over medium-low heat in a heavy-bottomed saucepan and put in the onion. Sauté until the onion becomes transparent. Add the garlic and bean purée. Now incorporate sauce, lime juice, cumin, flakes of red pepper, and salt or Vega-Sal. Once the soup is cooked through, turn the heat up a little and then turn it back down to the lowest level and let it boil for 30 to 45 minutes. Serve with a dollop of plain yogurt and a sprinkle of minced cilantro (or sour cream, if you prefer).

Nutrition:
- Protein: 18 g
- Fiber 25 g
- Dietary fiber: 13 g
- Available Carbohydrates: 13 g

409. Artichoke Soup

Difficulty: Easy
Preparation Time: 15 min
Cooking Time: 45 min
Servings: 6
Ingredients:
- Juice of ½ lemon
- 1 cup (240 ml) half-and-half
- ½ tsp guar or xanthan
- 0.9 L chicken broth, divided
- 1 can (14 ounces, or 410 g) quartered artichoke hearts, drained
- 1 garlic clove, crushed
- 2 stalks celery, finely chopped
- 1 small onion, finely chopped
- 4 tbsp (42 to 56 g) butter
- Salt or Vega-Sal
- Pepper

Directions:
1. Melt the butter in a big skillet, then sauté the celery, onion, and garlic over low to medium heat. Shake from time to time.
2. Drain the hearts of the artichoke and pick off any rough leaf pieces left on.
3. Placed the heart of the artichoke in a food processor with the S-blade in place. Add 1/2 cup (120 ml) of chicken broth and guar gum and strain until a fine purée is made from the artichokes. In a saucepan, scrape the artichoke mixture, add the remaining chicken broth, and boil over medium-high heat.
4. Stir the onion and celery into the artichoke mixture until tender. Whisk on the half-and-half when it comes to a boil. Take it back to a boil, push in the juice of a lemon and stir again. To taste, apply salt and pepper. You can eat this right now, hot, or you can eat it cold in the summer.

Nutrition:
- Carbs: 10 g
- Fiber: 3 g
- Protein: 4 g

410. Curried Pumpkin Soup

Difficulty: Easy
Preparation Time: 30 min
Cooking Time: 30 min
Servings: 6
Ingredients:
- 1 tsp curry powder
- ½ cup (120 ml) Carb Countdown dairy beverage
- 1½ cups (240 g) canned pumpkin
- 1 quart (960 ml) chicken broth
- 1 tbsp (14 g) butter
- 1 garlic clove
- ¼ cup (40 g) minced onion
- Salt and pepper to taste

Directions:
1. In a big saucepan, sauté the garlic and onion in butter, in a heavy-bottomed saucepan with medium-low heat until only softened. Put in the broth of the chicken and cook for half an hour.
2. Mix in the dairy beverage Carb Countdown, canned pumpkin, and Curry Powder. Adjust to a boil and cook softly for a further 15 minutes.
3. To taste, incorporate salt and pepper, and then eat.

Nutrition:
- Protein: 5 g
- Carbs: 7 g
- Dietary fiber: 2 g
- Usable carbs: 5 g

411. Cheesy Onion Soup

Difficulty: Easy
Preparation Time: 1 hour
Cooking Time: 1 hour
Servings: 4
Ingredients:
- ½ cup (120 ml) Carb Countdown dairy beverage
- 1 medium onion
- 1 quart (960 ml) beef broth
- ½ cup (120 ml) heavy cream
- Guar or xanthan (optional)
- 1½ cups (180 g) shredded sharp cheddar cheese
- Salt and pepper to taste

Directions:
1. In a large saucepan, add the beef broth and start heating it over a medium-high flame. Cut the paper-thin onion and apply it to the broth. Switch the heat down to low as the broth begins to boil and let the entire thing steam for 1 hour. You should do this ahead of time if you like; turn off the heat, let the entire thing cool, refrigerate it, and later do the rest. If you do this, before moving, lift the broth from heating again.
2. Stir in the cream and the dairy beverage Carb Timer softly. Now stir in the cheese, a little at a time, until all of it has melted. If you want to thicken with guar or xanthan, stir with a ladle or spoon instead of a whisk, you don't want to sever the onion threads.
3. Garnish with salt and pepper and serve.

Nutrition:
- Protein: 24 g
- Carbs: 8 g
- A trace of dietary fiber
- Usable carbs: 8 g

412. Cream of Potato Soup

Difficulty: Easy
Preparation Time: 1 hour
Cooking Time: 5 hours
Servings: 6
Ingredients:
- ½ cup (120 ml) Carb Countdown dairy beverage
- ½ cup (120 ml) heavy cream
- ½ cup (50 g) Ketones mix
- ½ cup (50 g) chopped onion
- ½ head cauliflower, chunked
- 1 quart (960 ml) chicken broth Guar or xanthan (optional)
- 5 scallions, sliced

Directions:
1. In your slow cooker, put cauliflower, broth, and onion. Close and set the slow cooker to low and run for about 4 to 5 hours.
2. We used a hand mixer to purée the soup right in the slow cooker; so alternatively, you should pass the cauliflower and onion into your blender or food processor, along with 1 cup (240 ml) of broth. Purée until entirely smooth, and then blend into the Ketatones, either way. If the cauliflower has been withdrawn from the slow cooker for purée, add the purée back in and whisk it back into the remaining broth.
3. Stir in the Carb Countdown and cream. If you believe it needs it, thicken it a little more with guar or xanthan.
4. To taste, apply salt and pepper and mix in the sliced scallions. Serve instantly hot or chill and serve as Vichyssoise.

Nutrition:
- Protein: 12 g
- Carbs: 13 g
- Dietary fiber: 6 g
- Usable carbs: 7 g

413. Swiss cheese and Broccoli Soup

Difficulty: Easy
Preparation Time: 10 min
Cooking Time: 1 hour
Servings: 6–8
Ingredients:
- Guar or xanthan
- 360 g shredded Swiss cheese
- 1 cup (240 ml) heavy cream
- 500 ml Carb Countdown dairy beverage
- 10 ounces (560 g) frozen chopped broccoli, thawed
- 28 ounces (400 ml) chicken broth
- 28 g butter
- 420 g minced onion

Directions:
1. Sauté the onion into the butter in a big, heavy-bottomed saucepan until it is transparent. Put the broccoli and the chicken broth in the pan and cook for 20 to 30 minutes until the broccoli is very soft.
2. Mix in the Countdown Carb and some cream. Bring it to a simmer again.
3. Now mix in the cheese, a little at a time, allowing each batch to melt before adding any more. Thicken a bit with guar or xanthan when all the cheese is melted if you think it needs it, and then serve.

Nutrition:
- Protein: 20 g
- Carbs: 7 g
- Dietary fiber: 2 g
- Usable carbs: 5 g

414. Tavern Soup

Difficulty: Easy
Preparation Time: 8–10 hours
Cooking Time: 1 hour
Servings: 8
Ingredients:
- 1/2 tsp hot pepper sauce
- 1 tsp salt or Vega-Sal
- 24 ounces (500 ml) light beer
- 900 g sharp cheddar cheese, shredded
- 1 tsp pepper
- 1/2 cup (30.4 g) chopped fresh parsley
- 1/2 cup (60 g) shredded carrot
- 1/2 cup (60 g) finely diced green bell pepper
- 1/2 cup (60 g) finely diced celery
- Guar or xanthan
- 3 L chicken broth

Directions:
1. Mix in your slow cooker celery, broth, green pepper, onion, parsley, and pepper. Close the slow cooker, set it to low, and let it steam for 6 to 8 hours (it won't hurt for a little longer).
2. To purée the vegetables in the slow cooker right there until the time is up, use a handheld blender to scoop them out with a slotted spoon, purée them in the blender, and add them to the slow cooker.
3. Now swirl a little at a time in the cheese until it's all melted. Add the hot pepper sauce, beer, salt, or Vega-Sal, and mix until the foaming ends.
4. To thicken the broth, use guar or xanthan until it is about sour cream thickness. Cover the pot again, turn it too heavy, and simmer for an additional 20 minutes before eating.

Nutrition:
- Protein: 18 g
- Carbs: 3 g
- A trace of dietary fiber
- Usable carbs: 3 g

415. Broccoli Blue Cheese Soup

Difficulty: Intermediate
Preparation Time: 1 hour
Cooking Time: 1 hour
Servings: 6–8
Ingredients:
- 1 cup (120 g) crumbled blue cheese
- ¼ cup (60 ml) heavy cream
- 1 pound (455 g) frozen broccoli, thawed
- 1½ quarts (1.4 L) chicken broth
- 1 cup (240 ml) Carb Countdown dairy beverage
- 1 turnip, peeled and diced
- 28 g butter
- 160 g chopped onion

Directions:
1. Sauté the onion in the butter over medium-low heat in a broad saucepan—you don't want it to tan.
2. Until the onion is soft and transparent, add the chicken broth and the turnip to your pot. Bring the blend to a boil and let it cook for 20 to 30 minutes over medium to low heat.
3. Put in the thawed broccoli and cook for the next 20 minutes.
4. With a slotted spoon, scoop the vegetables out and put them in a Mixer. A ladleful broth is added to the mix, and the blender runs until the vegetables are finely puréed. Shift the mixture back to your pot. Stir in the dairy beverage, the heavy cream, and the blue cheese. Simmer for the next 5 to 10 minutes, stirring periodically, and serve.

Nutrition:
- Protein: 14 g
- Carbs: 9 g
- Dietary fiber: 3 g
- Usable carbs: 6 g

416. **Cream of Mushroom Soup**

Difficulty: Easy
Preparation Time: 6 hours
Cooking Time: 1 1/2 hour
Servings: 5–7
Ingredients:
- ½ cup (120 g) light sour cream
- ½ cup (120 ml) heavy cream
- 1 quart (960 ml) chicken broth
- 28 g butter
- ¼ cup (25 g) chopped onion
- 8 ounces (225 g) mushrooms, sliced
- Guar or xanthan (optional)

Directions:
1. Sauté the onion and mushrooms in the butter in a large, heavy skillet until the mushrooms soften and change color. Move them to a slow cooker. Put in the broth. Cover your slow cooker, set it low and let it cook for 5 to 6 hours.
2. Scrape out the vegetables with a slotted spoon when the time is up, and stick them in your blender or any food processor.
3. Add in enough broth to help them quickly process and finely purée them. Put the puréed vegetables back into the slow cooker, using a rubber scraper to clean out any last pieces. Now whisk in the heavy cream and sour cream and apply to taste the salt and pepper. If you think it deserves it, thicken the sauce a little with guar or xanthan. Serve.

Nutrition:
- Protein: 6 g
- Carbs: 5 g
- Dietary fiber: 1 g
- Usable carbs: 4 g

417. **Olive Soup**

Difficulty: Medium
Preparation Time: 20 min
Cooking Time: 1 hour
Servings: 6–8
Ingredients:
- Pepper
- Salt or Vega-Sal
- ¼ cup (60 ml) dry sherry
- ½ tsp guar or xanthan
- 1 cup (100 g) minced black olives (You can buy cans of minced black olives.)
- 1 cup (240 ml) heavy cream
- 0.9 L chicken broth, divided

Directions:
1. Put 1/2 cup (120 ml) of the chicken broth with the guar gum in the blender and pulse for a few moments. Pour the remainder of the stock and the olives into a saucepan and add the blended mixture.
2. Heat and then whisk in the milk before simmering. Return to a boil, stir in the sherry, then apply salt and pepper to taste.

Nutrition:
- Carbs: 3,5 g
- Fiber: 1,1 g
- Usable carbs: 2,5 g
- Protein: 2,5 g

418. Wasabi Tuna Asian Salad

Difficulty: Easy
Preparation Time: 30 minutes
Cooking Time: 10 minutes
Servings: 1
Ingredients:
- 1 tsp Lime juice
- Non-stick cooking spray
- Dash of salt and pepper
- 1 tsp Wasabi paste
- 2 tsp Olive oil
- 1/2 cup Chopped or shredded cucumbers
- 1 cup Bok Choy stalks
- 8 oz. Raw tuna steak

Directions:
Fish:
1. Preheat your skillet to medium heat. Mix your wasabi and lime juice; coat the tuna steaks.
2. Use a non-stick cooking spray on your skillet for 10 seconds.
3. Put your tuna steaks on the skillet and cook over medium heat until you get the desired doneness.

Salad:
4. Slice the cucumber into match-stick tiny sizes. Cut the bok Choy into minute pieces. Toss gently with pepper, salt, and olive oil if you want.

Nutrition:
- Protein: 61 g
- Fiber: 1 g
- Cholesterol: 115 mg
- Saturated fats: 2 g
- Calories: 380

419. Lemon Greek Salad

Difficulty: Easy
Preparation Time: 25 minutes
Cooking Time: 25 minutes
Servings: 1
Ingredients:
- 140 oz. chicken breast
- 1 cup chopped cucumber
- 1 cup chopped orange/red bell pepper
- 1 cup wedged/sliced/chopped tomatoes
- 1/4 cup chopped olives
- 2 tbsp fresh parsley, finely chopped.
- 2 tbsp finely chopped red onion
- 5 tsp lemon juice
- 1 tsp olive oil
- 1 garlic clove, minced

Directions:
1. Preheat your grill to medium heat.
2. Grill the chicken and cook on each side until it is no longer pink or for 5 minutes.
3. Cut the chicken into tiny pieces. In your serving bowl, mix garlic, olives, and parsley. Whisk in olive oil (1 tsp) and lemon juice (4 tsp). Add onion, tomatoes, bell pepper, and cucumber.
4. Toss gently. Coat the ingredients with dressing. Add another tsp of lemon juice to taste. Divide the salad into two servings and put 6 oz chicken on top of each salad.

Nutrition:
- Protein: 56 g
- Fiber: 4 g
- Total carbs: 14 g
- Sodium: 280 mg
- Cholesterol: 145 mg
- Saturated fat: 2.5 g
- Total fat: 12 g
- Calories: 380

420. Broccoli Salad

Difficulty: Easy
Preparation Time: 5 minutes
Cooking Time: 25 minutes
Servings: 1
Ingredients:
- 1/3 tbsp sherry vinegar
- 1/2 cup olive oil
- 1/3 tsp fresh thyme, chopped
- 1/6 tsp Dijon mustard
- 1/6 tsp honey
- Salt to taste
- 1 1/3 cups broccoli florets
- 1/3 red onions
- 1/12 cup parmesan cheese shaved

Directions:
1. Mix the sherry vinegar, olive oil, thyme, mustard, honey, and salt in a bowl.
2. In a serving bowl, blend the broccoli florets and onions.
3. Drizzle the dressing on top.
4. Sprinkle with the pecans and parmesan cheese before serving.

Nutrition:
- Calories: 199
- Fat: 17.4 g
- Saturated fat: 2.9 g
- Carbohydrates: 7.5 g
- Fiber: 2.8 g
- Protein: 5.2 g

421. Potato Carrot Salad

Difficulty: Easy
Preparation Time: 15 minutes
Cooking Time: 10 minutes
Servings: 1
Ingredients:
- Water
- 1 potato, sliced into cubes
- 1/2 carrots, cut into cubes
- 1/6 tbsp milk
- 1/6 tbsp Dijon mustard
- 1/24 cup mayonnaise
- Pepper to taste
- 1/3 tsp fresh thyme, chopped
- 1/6 stalk celery, chopped
- 1/6 scallions, chopped
- 1/6 slice turkey bacon, cooked crispy and crumbled

Directions:
1. Fill your pot with water.
2. Place it over medium-high heat.
3. Boil the potatoes and carrots for 10 to 12 minutes or until tender.
4. Drain and let cool.
5. In a bowl, mix the milk, mustard, mayonnaise, pepper, and thyme.
6. Stir in the potatoes, carrots, and celery.
7. Coat evenly with the sauce.
8. Cover and refrigerate for 4 hours.
9. Top with the scallions and turkey bacon bits before serving.

Nutrition:
- Calories: 106
- Fat: 5.3 g
- Saturated fat: 1 g
- Carbohydrates: 12.6 g
- Fiber: 1.8 g
- Protein: 2 g

422. Marinated Veggie Salad

Difficulty: Easy
Preparation Time: 4 hours and 30 minutes
Cooking Time: 3 minutes
Servings: 1
Ingredients:
- 1 zucchini, sliced
- 4 tomatoes, sliced into wedges
- ¼ cup red onion, sliced thinly
- 1 green bell pepper, sliced
- 2 tbsp fresh parsley, chopped
- 2 tbsp red-wine vinegar
- 2 tbsp olive oil
- 1 garlic clove, minced
- 1 tsp dried basil
- 2 tbsp water
- Pine nuts, toasted and chopped

Directions:
1. In a bowl, combine the zucchini, tomatoes, red onion, green bell pepper, and parsley.
2. Pour the vinegar and oil into a glass jar with a lid.
3. Add the garlic, basil, and water.
4. Seal the jar and stir well to combine.
5. Pour the dressing into the vegetable mixture.
6. Cover the bowl.
7. Marinate in the refrigerator for 4 hours.
8. Garnish with the pine nuts before serving.

Nutrition:
- Calories: 65
- Fat: 4.7 g
- Saturated fat: 0.7 g
- Carbohydrates: 5.3 g
- Fiber: 1.2 g
- Protein: 0.9 g

423. Mediterranean Salad

Difficulty: Easy
Preparation Time: 20 minutes
Cooking Time: 5 minutes
Servings: 1
Ingredients:
- 1 tsp balsamic vinegar
- 1/2 tbsp basil pesto
- 1/2 cup lettuce
- 1/8 cup broccoli florets, chopped
- 1/8 cup zucchini, chopped
- 1/8 cup tomato, chopped
- 1/8 cup yellow bell pepper, chopped
- 1/2 tbsp feta cheese, crumbled

Directions:
1. Arrange the lettuce on a serving platter.
2. Top with broccoli, zucchini, tomato, and bell pepper.
3. In a bowl, mix the vinegar and pesto.
4. Drizzle the dressing on top.
5. Sprinkle the feta cheese.

Nutrition:
- Calories: 100
- Fat: 6 g
- Saturated fat: 1 g
- Carbohydrates: 7 g
- Protein: 4 g

424. Potato Tuna Salad

Difficulty: Easy
Preparation Time: 4 hours and 20 minutes
Cooking Time: 10 minutes
Servings: 1
Ingredients:
- 1 potato, peeled and sliced into cubes
- 1/12 cup plain yogurt
- 1/12 cup mayonnaise
- 1/6 garlic clove, crushed and minced
- 1/6 tbsp almond milk
- 1/6 tbsp fresh dill, chopped
- ½ tsp lemon zest
- Salt to taste
- 1 cup cucumber, chopped
- ¼ cup scallions, chopped
- ¼ cup radishes, chopped
- (9 oz.) canned tuna flakes
- 1/2 hard-boiled eggs, chopped
- 1 cups lettuce, chopped

Directions:
1. Fill your pot with water.
2. Add the potatoes and boil.
3. Cook for 15 minutes or till slightly tender.
4. Drain and let cool.
5. In a bowl, mix the yogurt, mayo, garlic, almond milk, fresh dill, lemon zest, and salt.
6. Stir in the potatoes, tuna flakes, and eggs.
7. Mix well.
8. Chill in the refrigerator for 4 hours.
9. Stir in the shredded lettuce before serving.

Nutrition:
- Calories: 243
- Fat: 9.9 g
- Saturated fat: 2 g
- Carbohydrates: 22.2 g
- Fiber: 4.6 g
- Protein: 17.5 g

425. High Protein Salad

Difficulty: Intermediate
Preparation Time: 5 minutes
Cooking Time: 5 minutes
Servings: 1
Ingredients:
Salad:
- 1(15 oz.) can green kidney beans
- 1/4 tbsp capers
- 1/4 handfuls arugula
- 1(15 oz.) can lentils

Dressing:
- 1/1 tbsp caper brine
- 1/1 tbsp tamari
- 1/1 tbsp balsamic vinegar
- 2/2 tbsp peanut butter
- 2/2 tbsp hot sauce
- 2/1 tbsp tahini

Directions:
For the dressing:
1. In a bowl, stir all the ingredients until they come together to form a smooth dressing.

For the salad:
2. Mix the beans, arugula, capers, and lentils. Top with the dressing and serve.

Nutrition:
- Calories: 205
- Fat: 2 g
- Protein: 13 g
- Carbs: 31 g
- Fiber: 17 g

426. Pea Salad

Difficulty: Easy
Preparation Time: 40 minutes
Cooking Time: 0 minutes
Servings: 1
Ingredients:
- 1/2 cup chickpeas, rinsed and drained
- 1/2 cups peas, divided
- Salt to taste
- 1 tbsp olive oil
- ½ cup buttermilk
- Pepper to taste
- 2 cups pea greens
- 1/2 carrots shaved
- 1/4 cup snow peas, trimmed

Directions:
1. Add the chickpeas and half of the peas to your food processor.
2. Season with salt.
3. Pulse until smooth. Set aside.
4. In a bowl, toss the remaining peas in oil, milk, salt, and pepper.
5. Transfer the mixture to your food processor.
6. Process until pureed.
7. Transfer this mixture to a bowl.
8. Arrange the pea greens on a serving plate.
9. Top with the shaved carrots and snow peas.
10. Stir in the pea and milk dressing.
11. Serve with the reserved chickpea hummus.

Nutrition:
- Calories: 214
- Fat: 8.6 g
- Saturated fat: 1.5 g
- Carbohydrates: 27.3 g
- Fiber: 8.4 g
- Protein: 8 g

427. Snap Pea Salad

Difficulty: Medium
Preparation Time: 1 hour
Cooking Time: 0 minutes
Servings: 1
Ingredients:
- 1/2 tbsp mayonnaise
- ¾ tsp celery seed
- ¼ cup cider vinegar
- 1/2 tsp yellow mustard
- 1/2 tbsp sugar
- Salt and pepper to taste
- 1 oz. radishes, sliced thinly
- 2 oz. sugar snap peas, sliced thinly

Directions:
1. In a bowl, combine the mayonnaise, celery seeds, vinegar, mustard, sugar, salt, and pepper.
2. Stir in the radishes and snap peas.
3. Refrigerate for 30 minutes.

Nutrition:
- Calories: 69
- Fat: 3.7 g
- Saturated fat: 0.6 g
- Carbohydrates: 7.1 g
- Fiber: 1.8 g
- Protein: 2 g

428. Cucumber Tomato Chopped Salad

Difficulty: Easy
Preparation Time: 15 minutes
Cooking Time: 0 minutes
Servings: 1
Ingredients:
- 1/4 cup light mayonnaise
- 1/2 tbsp lemon juice
- 1/2 tbsp fresh dill, chopped
- 1/2 tbsp chive, chopped
- 1/4 cup feta cheese, crumbled
- Salt and pepper to taste
- 1/2 red onion, chopped
- 1/2 cucumber, diced
- 1/2 radish, diced
- 1 tomato, diced
- 1 handful of Chives, chopped

Directions:
1. Combine the mayonnaise, lemon juice, fresh dill, chives, feta cheese, salt, and pepper in a bowl.
2. Mix well.
3. Stir in the onion, cucumber, radish, and tomatoes.
4. Coat evenly.
5. Garnish with the chopped chives.

Nutrition:
- Calories: 187
- Fat: 16.7 g
- Saturated fat: 4.1 g
- Carbohydrates: 6.7 g
- Fiber: 2 g
- Protein: 3.3 g

429. Zucchini Pasta Salad

Difficulty: Easy
Preparation Time: 4 minutes
Cooking Time: 0 minutes
Servings: 1
Ingredients:
- 1 tbsp olive oil
- 1/2 tsp Dijon mustard
- 1/3 tbsp red-wine vinegar
- 1/2 garlic clove, grated
- 2 tbsp fresh oregano, chopped
- 1/2 shallot, chopped
- ¼ tsp red pepper flakes
- 4 oz. zucchini noodles
- ¼ cup Kalamata olives pitted
- 1 cups cherry tomato, sliced in half
- ¾ cup parmesan cheese shaved

Directions:
1. Mix the olive oil, Dijon mustard, red wine vinegar, garlic, oregano, shallot, and red pepper flakes in a bowl.
2. Stir in the zucchini noodles.
3. Sprinkle on top with olives, tomatoes, and parmesan cheese.

Nutrition:
- Calories: 299
- Fat: 24.7 g
- Saturated fat: 5.1 g
- Carbohydrates: 11.6 g
- Fiber: 2.8 g
- Protein: 7 g

430. Egg Avocado Salad

Difficulty: Easy
Preparation Time: 10 minutes
Cooking Time: 0 minutes
Servings: 1
Ingredients:
- 1/2 avocado
- 1 hard-boiled egg, peeled and chopped
- 1/4 tbsp mayonnaise
- 1/4 tbsp freshly squeezed lemon juice ¼ cup celery, chopped
- 1/2 tbsp chives, chopped
- Salt and pepper to taste

Directions:
1. Add the avocado to a large bowl.
2. Mash the avocado using a fork.
3. Stir in the egg and mash the eggs.
4. Add the mayonnaise, lemon juice, celery, chives, salt, and pepper.
5. Chill in the refrigerator for at least 20 to 30 minutes before serving.

Nutrition:
- Calories: 224
- Fat: 18 g
- Saturated fat: 3.9 g
- Carbohydrates: 6.1 g
- Fiber: 3.6 g
- Protein: 10.6 g

431. Asian Cabbage Salad

Difficulty: Easy
Preparation Time: 10–15 minutes
Cooking Time: 2 minutes
Servings: 4–8
Ingredients:
- 4 cup green cabbage, shredded
- 1/4 cup red wine vinegar (no sugar added)
- 1 tbsp low sodium soy sauce
- 4 little spoon Stacey Hawkins Valencia Orange Oil (optional—can be made fat free simply by leaving out)
- 1 normal spoon Asian style seasoning
- 2 tsp lime juice

- 1/4 cup cilantro, chopped to taste with salt and pepper

Directions:
1. Combine shredded cabbage in a large bowl, green onions, cilantro, citrus dressing, and Asian seasoning (seeds removed, ground in a coffee grinder, or in a pestle and mortar, with a pestle); mix well. Chill in the refrigerator.

Nutrition:
- Calories: 99
- Protein: 4.13 g
- Fat: 4.53 g
- Carbohydrates: 12.47 g
- Calcium: 92 mg
- Magnesium: 35 mg
- Phosphorus: 95 mg

432. Tangy Kale Salad

Difficulty: Easy
Preparation Time: 20 minutes
Cooking Time: 6 minutes
Servings: 6
Ingredients:
- 1/2 cup olive oil
- 1/4 cup lemon juice
- 2 tbsp Dijon mustard
- 1 tbsp minced shallot
- 1 small garlic clove, finely minced
- 1/4 tsp salt, or more to taste ground black pepper to taste

Salad:
- 1 tsp olive oil
- 1/3 cup sliced almonds
- 1 bunch kale, center stems discarded and leaves thinly sliced 8 ounces Brussels sprouts, shredded
- 1 cup grated Pecorino Romano cheese

Directions:
1. Whisk together the lemon juice to create the dressing, olive oil, shallot, garlic, mustard, ¼ tsp salt, and pepper. Set aside.
2. To make the salad, heat the oil over medium-high heat in a large skillet. Add the almonds and cook, sometimes stirring, until the almonds are cooked. Almonds are ready. They are fragrant, and the oil is very aromatic for about 2 minutes. Transfer to a plate. Attach the skillet to the kale and cook until it begins to wilt and become colorful for about 4 minutes.
3. Add the Brussels sprouts, and reduce the heat to medium-low. Season with salt and pepper. Stuff the leaves with the cheese. Drizzle with the dressing.
4. Top with the almonds.

Nutrition:
- Calories: 193
- Protein: 1.74 g
- Fat: 19.11 g
- Carbohydrates: 5.56 g
- Calcium: 23 mg
- Magnesium: 14 mg

433. Crunchy Cauliflower Salad

Difficulty: Easy
Preparation Time: 10 minutes
Cooking Time: 10 minutes
Servings: 8
Ingredients:
- 4 cups cauliflower florets
- 1 tbsp (one capful) Stacey Hawkins Tuscan Fantasy Seasoning
- 1/4 cup apple cider vinegar

Directions:
1. In a wide bowl, position the cauliflower florets and coat them with a vinegar solution. Add Stacey Hawkins Tuscan Fantasy Seasoning and stir well. Let sit to allow the cauliflower to marinate for 10 minutes.
2. Preheat the oven to 450°F and Put a baking sheet on top of it—heavy-duty foil. On a baking sheet, put the marinated cauliflower and bake in the 450°F oven for 10–12 minutes. Remove and allow to cool.

Nutrition:
- Calories: 29
- Protein: 1.72 g
- Fat: 0.24 g
- Carbohydrates: 5.36 g
- Calcium: 20 mg
- Magnesium: 13 mg
- Phosphorus: 39 mg

434. Crisp Summer Cucumber Salad

Difficulty: Easy
Preparation Time: 15 minutes
Cooking Time: 0 minutes
Servings: 4
Ingredients:
- 4 cups sliced cucumbers (peels on or off—your choice)
- 2 tbsp apple cider vinegar
- 1/4 cup sliced white onion
- 2 tsp Stacey Hawkins Dash Desperation Seasoning

Directions:
1. Reserve some cucumber slices for garnish.
2. In a tub, mix up the rest of the ingredients.
3. Pour over the remaining cucumber slices and place in a pretty bowl.
4. Enable 15 minutes to sit down to absorb the flavor and serve.

Nutrition:
- Calories: 20
- Protein: 0.29 g
- Fat: 0.53 g
- Carbohydrates: 3.08 g
- Calcium: 3 mg
- Magnesium: 3 mg
- Phosphorus: 6 mg

AIR FRYER RECIPES

435. Air Fryer Italian Pork Chops

Difficulty: Easy
Preparation Time: 9 minutes
Cooking Time: 25 minutes
Servings: 2
Ingredients:
- 2 boneless pork loin chops, trimmed from fat (1 lean)
- ¼ tsp salt (1/8 condiment)
- 1 tsp Italian herb seasoning (1/8 condiment)

Directions:
1. Preheat the air fryer to 350°F for five minutes.
2. Wrap the bottom of the air fryer with foil.
3. Season the pork loin chops with spices and seasoning.
4. Place inside the air fryer basket and cook for 20 to 25 minutes.

Nutrition:
- Calories: 235
- Protein: 41 g
- Fat: 3g

436. Air Fried Riblets

Difficulty: Easy
Preparation Time: 9 minutes
Cooking Time: 25 minutes
Servings: 2
Ingredients:
- 1-pound pork riblets (1 lean)
- 1 tsp salt (1/8 condiment)
- 6 garlic cloves, minced (1/4 condiment)

Directions:
1. Preheat the air fryer to 350°F for five minutes.
2. Wrap the bottom of the air fryer with foil.
3. Season the pork riblets with salt and garlic.
4. Place inside the air fryer and cook for 20 to 25 minutes.

Nutrition:
- Calories: 288
- Protein: 39 g
- Fat: 12 g

437. Pork Tenderloin with Fried Bell Peppers

Difficulty: Medium
Preparation Time: 18 minutes
Cooking Time: 20 minutes
Servings: 4
Ingredients:
- 2 large bell peppers, seeded and julienned (1 green)
- 10 ounces Cremini mushrooms, diced (2 healthy fats)
- 1-pound pork tenderloin (1 lean)
- Salt and pepper to taste (1/8 condiment)

Directions:
1. Preheat the air fryer to 350°F for five minutes.
2. Line the bottom of the air fryer with foil.
3. Place all the ingredients in a bowl and toss to coat everything with the seasonings.
4. Place inside the air fryer basket and cook for 20 minutes.
5. Halfway through the cooking time, give the fryer basket a shake for even cooking.

Nutrition:
- Calories: 385
- Protein: 37 g
- Fat: 4.7 g

438. Air Fried Beef Jerky

Difficulty: Easy
Preparation Time: 11 minutes
Cooking Time: 15 minutes
Servings: 2
Ingredients:
- 12 ounces, sirloin beef, sliced (2 lean)
- 1 garlic clove, minced (1/2 condiment)
- Salt and pepper to taste (1/2 condiment)

Directions:
1. Preheat the air fryer to 350°F for five minutes.
2. Line the bottom of the air fryer with foil.

3. Place all the ingredients in a bowl and toss to coat the beef slices with the seasoning.
4. Place beef slices in the air fryer and cook for 15 minutes.

Nutrition:
- Calories: 333
- Protein: 35 g
- Fat: 14 g

439. <u>Air Fried Pot Roast</u>

Difficulty: Intermediate
Preparation Time: 12 minutes
Cooking Time: 60 minutes
Servings: 8
Ingredients:
- 4 pounds beef chuck roast (2 lean)
- Salt and pepper to taste (1/2 condiment)
- 5 garlic cloves, minced (1/2 condiment)
- 1 tsp thyme (1/2 green)

Directions:
1. Preheat the air fryer to 350°F for five minutes.
2. Line the bottom of the air fryer with foil.
3. Score the beef using a knife.
4. Season the pot roast with the seasoning.
5. Place inside the air fryer basket and cook for 60 minutes.

Nutrition:
- Calories: 420
- Protein: 61 g
- Fat: 16 g

440. <u>Mexican-Style Air Fryer Stuffed Chicken Breasts</u>

Difficulty: Easy
Preparation Time: 14 minutes
Cooking Time: 10 minutes
Servings: 2
Ingredients:
- 2 tsp olive oil (1/8 condiment)
- 1 chicken breast (skinless, boneless) (1 lean)
- 4 tsp chili powder, divided (1/8 condiment)
- 2 tsp chipotle flakes (1/8 condiment)
- 1/2 bell pepper, sliced (1/2 green)
- 2 tsp Mexican oregano (1/4 green)
- Salt and pepper, to taste (1/8 condiment)
- 4 tsp ground cumin, divided (1/8 condiment)
- 1/2 juice lime (1/8 condiment)
- 1 jalapeno pepper, sliced (1/4 green)

Directions:
1. In a bowl, add two tsp of cumin and two tsp of chili powder, mix well
2. Let the air fryer Preheat to 400°F
3. Pound the chicken breast until 1/4 inch of thickness remains.
4. In a bowl, mix the remaining chili powder, chipotle flakes, salt, oregano, remaining cumin, and pepper. Rub this spice mix all over the chicken.
5. Put half the bell pepper, jalapeno, and onion in the breast half. Roll the chicken around it and secure it with large toothpicks.
6. Add olive oil to breast rolls and coat in the cumin-chili mixture.
7. Add chicken breast to the air fryer and cook for six minutes.
8. Flip the breast rolls and cook for five minutes more until the chicken's temperature reaches 165°F.
9. Drizzle lime juice on top of breast rolls and serve hot.

Nutrition:
- Calories: 185.3
- Protein: 14 g
- Fat: 8.5 g

441. <u>Mixed Vegetables with Chicken</u>

Difficulty: Easy
Preparation Time: 11 minutes
Cooking Time: 20 minutes
Servings: 2
Ingredients:
- 4 cups Chicken breast, cubed pieces (1 lean)
- 1/2 zucchini chopped (1/2 green)
- 1 tbsp Italian seasoning (1/4 condiment)
- 1/2 cup Bell pepper chopped (1/2 green)
- 1 Garlic clove pressed (1/4 condiment)
- 1/2 cup Broccoli florets (1/2 green)
- 2 tbsp Olive oil (1/4 condiment)
- 1/2 tsp chili powder, garlic powder, pepper, salt, (1/4 condiment)

Directions:
1. Let the air fryer heat to 400°F and dice the vegetables
2. In a bowl, add the seasoning, oil, vegetables, and chicken and toss well
3. Place chicken and vegetables in the air fryer, and cook for ten minutes, tossing halfway through, and cook in batches.
4. Make sure the veggies are charred and the chicken is cooked through.
5. Serve hot.

Nutrition:
- Calories: 230
- Protein: 26 g
- Fat: 10 g

442. Low Carb Parmesan Chicken Meatballs

Difficulty: Easy
Preparation Time: 19 minutes
Cooking Time: 12 minutes
Servings: 20
Ingredients:
- 1/2 cup Pork rinds, ground (1 lean)
- 4 cups Ground chicken (2 lean)
- 1/2 cup Parmesan cheese, grated (1/2 healthy fat)
- 1 tsp Kosher salt (1/8 condiment)
- 1 tsp Garlic powder (1/8 condiment)
- 1 egg beaten (1/2 healthy fat)
- 1 tsp Paprika (1/8 condiment)
- 1/2 tsp Pepper (1/8 condiment)
- Breading (1/4 condiment)
- 1/2 cup Pork rinds, ground (1/2 healthy fat)

Directions:
1. Let the Air Fryer preheat to 400°F.
2. Add cheese, chicken, egg, and pepper, half cup of pork rinds, garlic, salt, and paprika in a big mixing ball. Mix well into a dough, make into 1 and half-inch balls.
3. Coat the meatballs in pork rinds (ground).
4. Oil sprays the air fry basket and add meatballs in one even layer.
5. Let it cook for 12 minutes at 400°F, flipping once halfway through.
6. Serve with salad greens.

Nutrition:
- Calories: 240
- Fat: 10 g
- Protein: 20 g

443. Sriracha-honey Chicken Wings

Difficulty: Easy
Preparation Time: 21 minutes
Cooking Time: 15 minutes
Servings: 2
Ingredients:
- 1 1/2 tbsp Soy sauce (1/4 condiment)
- 4 cups Chicken wings (2 lean)
- 2 tbsp Sriracha sauce (1/4 condiment)
- 1 tbsp (Butter: 1/2 healthy fat)
- 1/2 cup honey (1/2 healthy fat)
- Juice of half lime (1/4 condiment)
- Scallions cilantro, and chives for garnish (1/4 green)

Directions:
1. Let the air fryer preheat to 360°F.
2. Put the chicken wings in an air fryer basket, cook for half an hour, flip the wings every seven minutes, and cook thoroughly.
3. Meanwhile, in a saucepan, add all the ingredients of the sauce and simmer for three minutes.
4. Take out the chicken wings and coat them in sauce well.
5. Garnish with scallions. Serve with a microgreen salad.

Nutrition:
- Calories: 207
- Protein: 22 g
- Fat: 15 g

444. Orange Chicken Wings

Difficulty: Medium
Preparation Time: 19 minutes
Cooking Time: 14 minutes
Servings: 2
Ingredients:
- 1 tbsp Honey (1/2 healthy fat)
- Chicken Wings, Six pieces (3 lean)
- 1 orange zest, and juice (1/2 healthy fat)
- 1.5 tbsp Worcestershire Sauce (1/4 condiment)
- Black pepper to taste (1/4 condiment)
- Herbs (sage, rosemary, oregano, parsley, basil, thyme, and mint)

Directions:
1. Wash and pat dry the chicken wings
2. In a bowl, add chicken wings, and pour zest and orange juice
3. Add the rest of the ingredients and rub on chicken wings. Let it marinate for at least half an hour.
4. Let the Air fryer preheat at 180°C
5. In an aluminum foil, wrap the marinated wings and put them in an air fryer, and cook for 20 minutes at 180°C
6. After 20 minutes, remove the aluminum foil and brush the sauce over the wings and cook for 15 minutes more. Then again, brush the sauce and cook for another ten minutes.
7. Take out from the air fryer and serve with salad greens.

Nutrition:
- Calories: 271
- Protein: 29 g
- Fat: 15 g

445. Air Fryer Catfish with Cajun Seasoning

Difficulty: Easy
Preparation Time: 5 minutes
Cooking Time: 27 minutes
Servings: 4
Ingredients:
- 3 tsp Cajun seasoning (1/2 condiment)
- 3/4 cup Cornmeal (1/2 healthy fat)
- 4 catfish fillets (2 lean)

Directions:
1. In a zip lock bag, add Cajun seasoning and cornmeal
2. Wash and pat dry the catfish fillets. Add them to the zip lock bag.
3. Coat well the fillets with seasoning
4. Put catfish fillets in the air fryer and cook for 15 minutes at 390°F, turn fillets halfway through. To get a golden color on the fillets, cook for five more minutes.
5. Serve with lemon wedges and spicy tartar sauce.

Nutrition:
- Calories: 324
- Fat: 14 g
- Protein: 26.3 g

446. Air Fryer Sushi Roll

Difficulty: Easy
Preparation Time: 91 minutes
Cooking Time: 9 minutes
Servings: 3
Ingredients:
For the Kale Salad:
- 1/2 tsp Rice vinegar (1/8 condiment)
- 1 1/2 cups Chopped kale (1/2 green)
- 1/8 tsp Garlic powder (1/8 condiment)
- 1 tbsp Sesame seeds (1/4 healthy fat)
- 3/4 tsp Toasted sesame oil (1/8 condiment)
- 1/4 tsp ground ginger (1/8 condiment)
- 3/4 tsp Soy sauce (1/8 condiment)

Sushi Rolls:
- Half avocado—sliced (1/2 healthy fat)
- Cooked Sushi Rice—cooled (1 healthy fat)
- Half cup Whole wheat breadcrumbs (1/2 healthy fat)
- 3 sheets Sushi

Directions:
Make the Kale Salad
1. In a bowl, add vinegar, garlic powder, kale, soy sauce, sesame oil, and ground ginger. With your hands, mix with sesame seeds and set them aside.

Sushi Rolls
1. Lay a sheet of sushi on a flat surface. With damp fingertips, add a tbsp of rice, and

spread it on the sheet. Cover the sheet with rice, leaving half-inch space at one end.
2. Add kale salad with avocado slices. Roll up the sushi, and use water if needed.
3. Add the breadcrumbs to a bowl. Coat the sushi roll with Sriracha Mayo, then in breadcrumbs.
4. Add the rolls to the air fryer. Cook for ten minutes at 390°F, and shake the basket halfway through.
5. Take them out from the fryer, and let them cool, then cut with a sharp knife.
6. Serve with soy sauce.

Nutrition:
- Calories: 369
- Fat: 13.9 g
- Protein: 26 g

447. Air Fryer Garlic-Lime Shrimp Kebabs

Difficulty: Easy
Preparation Time: 5 minutes
Cooking Time: 19 minutes
Servings: 2
Ingredients:
- 1 lime (1/4 condiment)
- 1 cup raw shrimp (1 lean)
- 1/8 tsp salt (1/4 condiment)
- 1 garlic clove (1/4 condiment)
- Freshly ground black pepper (1/4 condiment)

Directions:
1. In water, let wooden skewers soak for 20 minutes.
2. Let the Air fryer preheat to 350°F.
3. In a bowl, mix shrimp, minced garlic, lime juice, kosher salt, and pepper
4. Add shrimp on skewers.
5. Place skewers in the air fryer, and cook for 8 minutes. Turn halfway over.
6. Top with cilantro and your favorite dip.

Nutrition:
- Calories: 76
- Protein: 13 g
- Fat: 9 g

448. Fish Finger Sandwich

Difficulty: Easy
Preparation Time: 10 minutes
Cooking Time: 9 minutes
Servings: 4
Ingredients:
- 1 tbsp Greek yogurt (1/2 healthy fat)
- 4 Cod fillets, without skin (2 lean)
- 2 tbsp Flour (1/4 healthy fat)
- 5 tbsp Whole-wheat breadcrumbs (1/4 healthy fat)
- Kosher salt and pepper, to taste (1/4 condiment)
- 10–12 Capers (1/2 healthy fat)
- Lemon juice (1/4 condiment)

Directions:
1. Let the air fryer preheat.
2. Sprinkle kosher salt and pepper on the cod fillets, and coat in flour, then in breadcrumbs
3. Spray the fryer basket with oil. Put the cod fillets in the basket.
4. Cook for 15 minutes at 200°C.
5. In the meantime, blend with Greek yogurt, lemon juice, and capers until well combined.
6. On a bun, add cooked fish with pea puree. Add lettuce and tomato.

Nutrition:
- Calories: 240
- Fat: 12 g
- Protein: 20 g

449. Healthy Air Fryer Tuna Patties

Difficulty: Easy
Preparation Time: 15 minutes
Cooking Time: 11 minutes
Servings: 10
Ingredients:
- 1/2 cup whole-wheat breadcrumbs (1/4 healthy fat)
- 4 cups fresh tuna, diced (2 lean)
- Lemon zest (1/4 condiment)
- 1 tbsp lemon juice: (1/4 condiment)
- 1 egg (1/4 healthy fat)
- 3 tbsp grated parmesan cheese (1/4 healthy fat)

- 1 chopped stalk celery (1 green)
- 1/2 tsp garlic powder: (1/4 condiment)
- 1/2 tsp dried herbs (1/4 green)
- Salt to taste (1/8 condiment)
- Freshly ground black pepper (1/8 condiment)

Directions:
1. In a bowl, add lemon zest, bread crumbs, salt, pepper, celery, eggs, dried herbs, lemon juice, garlic powder, parmesan cheese, and onion. Mix everything. Then add in tuna gently. Shape into patties. If the mixture is too loose, cool in the refrigerator.
2. Add air fryer baking paper to the air fryer basket. Spray the baking paper with cooking spray.
3. Spray the patties with oil.
4. Cook for ten minutes at 360°F. Turn the patties halfway over.
5. Serve with lemon slices and microgreens.

Nutrition:
- Calories: 214
- Fat: 15 g
- Protein: 22 g

450. Cheese Broccoli Fritters

Difficulty: Easy
Preparation Time: 10 minutes
Cooking Time: 30 minutes
Servings: 4
Ingredients:
- 2 eggs, lightly beaten (1/2 healthy fat)
- 3 cups broccoli florets, cooked & mashed (1 lean)
- 2 cups cheddar cheese (1/2 healthy fat)
- 1/4 cup almond flour (1/4 condiment)
- 2 garlic cloves, minced (1/4 condiment)
- Pepper (1/4 condiment)
- Salt (1/4 condiment)

Directions:
1. Mix all the ingredients into the bowl.
2. Make patties from the mixture and place them into the basket and cook at 350°F for 15 minutes.
3. Turn patties and cook for 15 minutes more.
4. Serve and enjoy.

Nutrition:
- Calories: 285
- Fat: 21 g
- Protein: 18 g

451. Air Fryer Bell Peppers

Difficulty: Medium
Preparation Time: 10 minutes
Cooking Time: 8 minutes
Servings: 3
Ingredients:
- ¼ tsp onion powder (1/4 condiment)
- 3 cups bell peppers, cut into pieces (1 green)
- 1 tsp olive oil (1/2 condiment)
- 1/4 tsp garlic powder (1/4 condiment)

Directions:
1. Mix all the ingredients into a large bowl and toss well.
2. Transfer bell peppers into the air fryer basket and cook at 360°F for 8 minutes. Stir halfway through.
3. Serve and enjoy.

Nutrition:
- Calories: 52
- Fat: 2 g
- Protein: 1.2 g

452. Air Fried Tasty Eggplant

Difficulty: Easy
Preparation Time: 10 minutes
Cooking Time: 12 minutes
Servings: 2
Ingredients:
- 1 eggplant, cut into cubes (1 green)
- 1/4 tsp oregano (1/4 green)
- 1 tbsp olive oil (1/2 condiment)
- 1/2 tsp garlic powder (1/4 condiment)
- 1/4 tsp chili powder (1/4 condiment)

Directions:
1. Incorporate all the ingredients into the huge bowl and toss well.
2. Transfer eggplant into the air fryer basket and cook at 390°F for 12 minutes. Stir halfway through.
3. Serve and enjoy.

Nutrition:
- Calories: 120
- Fat: 7 g
- Protein: 2 g

453. Asian Green Beans

Difficulty: Easy
Preparation Time: 10 minutes
Cooking Time: 10 minutes
Servings: 2
Ingredients:
- 8 oz. green beans (1 green)
- 1 tbsp tamari (1/2 condiment)
- 1 tsp sesame oil (1/2 condiment)

Directions:
1. Mix all the ingredients into the big bowl and toss well.
2. Add green beans into the air fryer basket and cook at 400°F for 10 minutes.
3. Serve and enjoy.

Nutrition:
- Calories: 60
- Fat: 2 g
- Protein: 3 g

454. Spicy Asian Brussels Sprouts

Difficulty: Intermediate
Preparation Time: 10 minutes
Cooking Time: 15 minutes
Servings: 4
Ingredients:
- 1 lb. Brussels sprouts, cut in half (1 green)
- 1 tbsp gochujang (1/2 condiment)
- 1 1/2 tbsp olive oil (1/4 condiment)
- 1/2 tsp salt (1/4 condiment)

Directions:
1. In a bowl, mix olive oil, gochujang, and salt.
2. Add Brussels sprouts into the bowl and toss until well coated.
3. Add Brussels sprouts into the air fryer basket and cook at 360°F for 15 minutes.
4. Serve and enjoy.

Nutrition:
- Calories: 94
- Fat: 5 g
- Protein: 4 g

455. Taco Salad

Preparation Time: 5 minutes.
Cooking Time: 0 minutes.
Servings: 2
Ingredients:
- 5 ounces ground turkey
- 1 tbsp taco seasoning
- 2 tbsp salsa
- 1/2 cup romaine lettuce
- 1/2 cup iceberg lettuce
- 1/2 cup diced tomatoes
- 1 tbsp water

Directions:
1. Sauté turkey with taco seasoning in a skillet until golden brown.
2. Transfer to a salad bowl and stir in salsa, lettuce, tomatoes, and water.
3. Mix well and serve.

Serving Suggestion:
4. Serve this salad with grilled chicken.

Variation Tip:
5. Drizzle black pepper ground on top before serving.

Nutrition:
- Calories: 345
- Fat: 9 g
- Sodium: 48 mg
- Carbs: 14 g
- Fiber: 1 g
- Sugar: 2 g
- Protein: 20 g

456. Yogurt Trail Mix Bars

Preparation Time: 15 minutes.
Cooking Time: 0 minutes.
Servings: 4
Ingredients:
- 2 cups Greek yogurt
- ½ cup fruit
- ½ cup almonds, chopped
- ¾ cup granola
- ¼ cup chocolate chips

Directions:
1. Mix yogurt with fruit, almonds, granola, and chocolate chips in a bowl.
2. Spread this mixture in a shallow tray and freeze for 1 hour.
3. Cut the mixture into bars.
4. Serve.

Serving Suggestion:
5. Serve these bars with a berry compote.

Variation Tip:
6. Pour melted chocolates on top and then slice to serve.

Nutrition:
- Calories: 204
- Fat: 3 g
- Sodium: 216 mg
- Carbs: 17 g
- Fiber: 3 g
- Sugar: 4 g
- Protein: 11 g

457. Curried Tuna Salad

Preparation Time: 15 minutes.
Cooking Time: 0 minutes.
Servings: 2
Ingredients:
- 2 cans tuna, drained
- ¼ cup hummus
- ¼ cup avocado, smashed
- ½ cup apple, chopped
- ¼ cup onion, diced
- 1 tbsp lemon juice
- 1 tsp curry powder
- 1/2 tsp dry mustard powder

Directions:
1. Mix tuna with the rest of the ingredients in a salad bowl.
2. Serve fresh.

Serving Suggestion:
3. Serve this salad with grilled shrimp.

Variation Tip:
4. Drizzle shredded coconut on top before serving.

Nutrition:
- Calories: 280
- Fat: 9 g
- Sodium: 318 mg
- Carbs: 19 g
- Fiber: 5 g
- Sugar: 3 g
- Protein: 17 g

MEAL PLAN 5&1

Week 1

DAY	BREAKFAST & LUNCH	DINNER
1	SWEET CASHEW CHEESE SPREAD LEAN AND GREEN SMOOTHIE 2 STUFFED MUSHROOMS FLAVORFUL KETO TACO SOUP TACO CASSEROLE	WARM CHORIZO CHICKPEA SALAD
2	CHOCOLATE CAKE FRIES YOGURT CEREAL BARK CRUNCH SANDWICH COOKIES MINI MAC IN A BOWL ALKALINE BLUEBERRY MUFFINS	FENNEL WILD RICE RISOTTO
3	BROCCOLI EGG BAKE SCRAMBLED PESTO EGGS YOGURT GARLIC CHICKEN BLUE CHEESE CHICKEN WEDGES MEATBALLS CURRY	GREEK STYLE QUESADILLAS
4	ZUCCHINI BREAKFAST BARS JALAPENO BREAKFAST CASSEROLE KETO CHEESY BROCCOLI SOUP BAKED CHICKEN FAJITAS SAUTÉD CRISPY ZUCCHINI	PROSCIUTTO WRAPPED MOZZARELLA BALLS
5	LEAN AND GREEN SMOOTHIE 1 ALKALINE BLUEBERRY SPELT PANCAKES COCONUT PANCAKES CRAB CAKES AMAZING LOW-CARB SHRIMP LETTUCE WRAPS.	QUINOA WITH VEGETABLES
6	ZUCCHINI BACON BAKE COTTAGE CHEESE HOTCAKE QUICK KETO BLT CHICKEN SALAD MASHED GARLIC TURNIPS 'I LOVE BACON'	TOMATO FISH BAKE
7	EGG & BACON CUPS CINNAMON COCONUT PORRIDGE LEMONGRASS PRAWNS KETO ZUCCHINI PIZZA EASY KETO CHICKEN SOUP	CHICKEN BROCCOLI SALAD WITH AVOCADO DRESSING

Week 2

DAY	BREAKFAST & LUNCH	DINNER
1	CHOCOLATE WHOOPIE PIES PIZZA HACK SAUSAGE EGG OMELET CREAMY LOW CARB CREAM OF MUSHROOM SOUP YUMMY KETO MUSHROOM ASPARAGUS FRITTATA	BAKED BEEF ZUCCHINI
2	MUSHROOM & SPINACH OMELET WHOLE-WHEAT BLUEBERRY MUFFINS ASPARAGUS & CRABMEAT FRITTATA OMEGA-3 SALAD DELICIOUS INSTANT POT KETO BUFFALO CHICKEN SOUP	STUFFED BELL PEPPERS WITH QUINOA
3	EASY CHEESE EGG BAKE CHICKEN CHEESE QUICHE HONEY GLAZED CHICKEN DRUMSTICKS LOW CARB BLACK BEANS CHILI CHICKEN QUICK KETO BLT CHICKEN SALAD	JARLSBERG LUNCH OMELET
4	HOT CHOCOLATE YOGURT COOKIE DOUGH BROWNIE PEANUT BUTTER PUDDING PEANUT BUTTER COOKIES CAULIFLOWER BREAKFAST CASSEROLE	FIERY JALAPENO POPPERS
5	VANILLA SHAKE PEPPERMINT MOCHA CHOCOLATE FRAPPE CARAMEL CRUNCH PARFAIT FUDGE BALLS	CHEDDAR BACON BURST
6	GREEN BEAN CASSEROLE CABBAGE AND RADISHES MIX SPINACH AND ARTICHOKES SAUTÉ HERBED RADISH SAUTÉ BOK CHOY AND BUTTER SAUCE	MEDITERRANEAN BURRITO
7	KALE AND WALNUTS BERRY MOJITO COCONUT SMOOTHIE CHOCOLATE SHAKE VANILLA FRAPPE	GARLIC CHICKEN BALLS

Week 3

DAY	BREAKFAST & LUNCH	DINNER
1	KALE CHIPS GREEN BEANS TIRAMISU SHAKE CARAMEL MACCHIATO FRAPPE PUMPKIN SPICED LATTE	GRILLED SALMON WITH PINEAPPLE SALSA
2	EGGNOG CHERRY MOCHA POPSICLES BROWNIE PUDDING MINT COOKIES SNICKERDOODLES	MOZZARELLA STICKS
3	CHOCOLATE HAYSTACKS GLUTEN-FREE PANCAKES HEMP SEED PORRIDGE LEAN AND GREEN CHICKEN PESTO PASTA OPEN-FACE EGG SANDWICHES WITH CILANTRO-JALAPEÑO SPREAD	HERBED ROASTED CHICKEN BREASTS
4	CRUNCHY QUINOA MEAL CHEESY SCRAMBLED TOFU CHARD OMELET DEVIL EGGS ANCHO TILAPIA ON CAULIFLOWER RICE	LIGHT PAPRIKA MOUSSAKA
5	TURKEY CAPRESE MEATLOAF CUPS BACON-WRAPPED ASPARAGUS QUICK HEALTHY AVOCADO TUNA SALAD QUICK KETO ROASTED TOMATO SOUP TASTY LOW-CARB CUCUMBER SALAD.	SWEET POTATO BACON MASH
6	PLANT-POWERED PANCAKES BISCUIT PIZZA CREAMY LOW CARB ZUCCHINI ALFREDO GRILLED HAM & CHEESE RICED CAULIFLOWER & CURRY CHICKEN	DILL RELISH ON WHITE SEA BASS
7	CHOCOLATE BERRY PARFAIT CHOCOLATE CAKE FRIES CHOCOLATE CRUNCH COOKIES GINGERSNAP COOKIES WHOLE-WHEAT BLUEBERRY MUFFINS	CHICKEN & TURKEY MEATLOAF

Week 4

DAY	BREAKFAST & LUNCH	DINNER
1	SHAKE CAKE FUELING CASHEW YOGURT BOWL CHICKEN CHEESE QUICHE PROSCIUTTO SPINACH SALAD PORK TACO BAKE	PAN-FRIED SALMON
2	FRENCH TOAST STICKS PEANUT BUTTER BITES MINI ZUCCHINI BITES WALNUT CRUNCH BANANA BREAD BISCUIT PIZZA	GRANDMA'S RICE
3	CHOCOLATE COCONUT PIE OATMEAL COOKIES ZUCCHINI BACON BAKE SPINACH CHICKEN DELICIOUS LOW CARB CHICKEN CAESAR SALAD	BAKED TUNA WITH ASPARAGUS
4	CLASSIC LOW CARB COBB SALAD LASAGNA SPAGHETTI SQUASH 'OH SO GOOD' SALAD LEMON DILL TROUT PORK WITH VEGGIES	GARLICKY TOMATO CHICKEN CASSEROLE
5	CHIA SEED PUDDING SNICKERDOODLES BROWNIE BITES SPINACH PIE PESTO ZUCCHINI NOODLES	MARINATED CHICKEN BREASTS
6	PARMESAN ZUCCHINI ROUNDS SPINACH AND ARTICHOKES SAUTÉ ROASTED TOMATOES TURMERIC MUSHROOM SHAMROCK SHAKE	CUCUMBER CONTAINER WITH SPICES AND GREEK YOGURT
7	ZUCCHINI SPAGHETTI CORIANDER ARTICHOKES BALSAMIC CABBAGE PUMPKIN FRAPPE BROWNIE PEANUT BUTTER PUDDING	CHICKEN GOULASH

MEAL PLAN 4&2&1

Week 1

DAY	4 FUELING HACKS	2 LEAN AND GREEN MEALS	1 SNACK
1	ZUCCHINI SPAGHETTI BALSAMIC CABBAGE BOK CHOY AND BUTTER SAUCE PEPPERMINT MOCHA	MEDITERRANEAN CHICKPEA SALAD MOZZARELLA STICKS	STUFFED AVOCADO
2	TIRAMISU SHAKE VANILLA FRAPPE CHOCOLATE COCONUT PIE CHIA SEED PUDDING	YOGURT GARLIC CHICKEN CUCUMBER CONTAINER WITH SPICES AND GREEK YOGURT	AVOCADO TACO BOATS
3	CHERRY MOCHA POPSICLES BROWNIE PUDDING YOGURT CEREAL BARK MINT COOKIES	STUFFED MUSHROOMS LOW CARB BLACK BEANS CHILI CHICKEN	MARINATED EGGS
4	CHOCOLATE BERRY PARFAIT FUDGE BALLS SANDWICH COOKIES CHOCOLATE WHOOPIE PIES	DELICIOUS LOW CARB CHICKEN CAESAR SALAD MEATBALLS CURRY	VEGGIE FRITTERS
5	HOT CHOCOLATE CHOCOLATE COCONUT PIE CHIA SEED PUDDING PEANUT BUTTER COOKIES	ZUCCHINI SALMON SALAD GREEK ROASTED FISH	EGGPLANT DIP
6	SHAMROCK SHAKE PUMPKIN SPICED LATTE HOT CHOCOLATE FRENCH TOAST STICKS	WILD RICE PRAWN SALAD SEAFOOD PAELLA	CREAMY SPINACH AND SHALLOTS DIP
7	GREEN BEAN CASSEROLE SPINACH AND ARTICHOKES SAUTÉ ROASTED TOMATOES BERRY MOJITO	LAMB STUFFED AVOCADO CREAMY PENNE	GARLIC KALE

Week 2

DAY	4 FUELING HACKS	2 LEAN AND GREEN MEALS	1 SNACK
1	PARMESAN ZUCCHINI ROUNDS KALE CHIPS CORIANDER ARTICHOKES TURMERIC MUSHROOM	MONKEY SALAD BACON & CHICKEN PATTIES	CHICKEN ENCHILADA BAKE
2	GREEN BEANS BERRY MOJITO PEPPERMINT MOCHA PUMPKIN SPICED LATTE	MEDITERRANEAN BURRITO MU SHU LUNCH PORK	AVOCADO DIP
3	FRENCH TOAST STICKS GINGERSNAP COOKIES SNICKERDOODLES CHOCOLATE HAYSTACKS	CHICKEN CACCIATORE SEAFOOD PAELLA	GOAT CHEESE AND CHIVES SPREAD
4	CHOCOLATE CAKE FRIES PEANUT BUTTER BITES OATMEAL COOKIES CRUNCH SANDWICH COOKIES	LAMB STUFFED AVOCADO GREEK ROASTED FISH	GREEN BEANS RICE
5	CARAMEL MACCHIATO FRAPPE EGGNOG BROWNIE PEANUT BUTTER PUDDING CHOCOLATE CRUNCH COOKIES	JALAPENO LENTIL BURGERS STUFFED BELL PEPPERS WITH QUINOA	CELERY AND GREEN BEANS MIX
6	CHOCOLATE SHAKE PUMPKIN FRAPPE YOGURT COOKIE DOUGH CARAMEL CRUNCH PARFAIT	ZUCCHINI SALMON SALAD CHICKEN CACCIATORE	PARMESAN ASPARAGUS
7	KALE AND WALNUTS COCONUT SMOOTHIE VANILLA SHAKE CHOCOLATE FRAPPE	LEMONGRASS PRAWNS DELICIOUS LOW CARB CHICKEN CAESAR SALAD	SPICY RED CABBAGE

Week 3

DAY	4 FUELING HACKS	2 LEAN AND GREEN MEALS	1 SNACK
1	CABBAGE AND RADISHES MIX GREEN BEANS HERBED RADISH SAUTÉ CHOCOLATE FRAPPE	FLAVORFUL KETO TACO SOUP GRILLED HAM & CHEESE	STUFFED AVOCADO
2	PUMPKIN FRAPPE CHIA SEED PUDDING OATMEAL COOKIES SANDWICH COOKIES	MEATBALLS CURRY LAMB STUFFED AVOCADO	PESTO CRACKERS
3	CHOCOLATE BERRY PARFAIT OATMEAL COOKIES SANDWICH COOKIES BROWNIE BITES	FENNEL WILD RICE RISOTTO GREEK STYLE QUESADILLAS	CHILI MANGO AND WATERMELON SALSA
4	ROASTED TOMATOES COCONUT SMOOTHIE VANILLA FRAPPE YOGURT COOKIE DOUGH	MEDITERRANEAN BURRITO MU SHU LUNCH PORK	GREEK TUNA SALAD BITES
5	CABBAGE AND RADISHES MIX SPINACH AND ARTICHOKES SAUTÉ KALE AND WALNUTS CHERRY MOCHA POPSICLES	MONKEY SALAD CHICKEN GOULASH	DIFFICULTY: EASY
6	KALE CHIPS GREEN BEANS CHOCOLATE SHAKE CHOCOLATE BERRY PARFAIT	BLUE CHEESE CHICKEN WEDGES GREEK STYLE QUESADILLAS	OLIVES AND CHEESE STUFFED TOMATOES
7	TIRAMISU SHAKE CHOCOLATE COCONUT PIE PEANUT BUTTER BITES SANDWICH COOKIES	HONEY GLAZED CHICKEN DRUMSTICKS EASY KETO CHICKEN SOUP	WHITE BEAN DIP

Week 4

DAY	4 FUELING HACKS	2 LEAN AND GREEN MEALS	1 SNACK
1	VANILLA SHAKE PEPPERMINT MOCHA CARAMEL MACCHIATO FRAPPE BROWNIE PUDDING	CHARD OMELET STUFFED MUSHROOMS	TASTY ONION AND CAULIFLOWER DIP
2	YOGURT COOKIE DOUGH PEANUT BUTTER BITES CHOCOLATE CRUNCH COOKIES GINGERSNAP COOKIES	WALNUT CRUNCH BANANA BREAD CHEESY SCRAMBLED TOFU	CHICKEN AND MUSHROOMS
3	GREEN BEAN CASSEROLE CORIANDER ARTICHOKES BALSAMIC CABBAGE COCONUT SMOOTHIE	OPEN-FACE EGG SANDWICHES WITH CILANTRO-JALAPEÑO SPREAD CREAMY LOW CARB ZUCCHINI ALFREDO	PUMPKIN MUFFINS
4	COCONUT SMOOTHIE CHOCOLATE SHAKE CHOCOLATE FRAPPE EGGNOG	MASHED GARLIC TURNIPS PORK WITH VEGGIES	PREPARATION TIME:
5	TURMERIC MUSHROOM HOT CHOCOLATE BROWNIE PUDDING FUDGE BALLS	PESTO ZUCCHINI NOODLES JALAPENO LENTIL BURGERS	TOMATO SALSA
6	PARMESAN ZUCCHINI ROUNDS TURMERIC MUSHROOM SHAMROCK SHAKE CARAMEL MACCHIATO FRAPPE	LAMB STUFFED AVOCADO WILD RICE PRAWN SALAD	HUMMUS WITH GROUND LAMB
7	CABBAGE AND RADISHES MIX BALSAMIC CABBAGE TURMERIC MUSHROOM COCONUT SMOOTHIE	WARM CHORIZO CHICKPEA SALAD CREAMY PENNE	CUCUMBER ROLLS

CONCLUSION

A diet is the practice of eating food in a certain way. The word can also mean an individual's usual and customary diet. The recommended daily intake of calories, protein, fat, and carbohydrates varies depending on factors such as age and gender.

There are many benefits to taking up the Lean & Green Diet which include better digestion, more energy from food, weight loss, lower risk of obesity/diabetes, and more. Some popular benefits would be that a person on this diet will lose weight quickly which will allow them to tone their body and improve their appearance which will make it easier for people who may be shy about revealing their skin condition(s). They will be able to eat more foods that are healthy and fit for their current dietary lifestyle. Within the next few years, there will be more studies done on the effects of this diet upon individuals' bodies and many benefits could be discovered.

Lean & Green Diet can also be used as a supplement or a prescription to help with weight loss or other issues. It can provide benefits such as less caused by diabetes, heart disease, asthma, cholesterol, cancer, and other conditions. It also avoids fat oxidation which is a side effect of high levels of Carbohydrates: which are said to cause obesity. A less likely benefit is that this diet can also help someone diagnosed with diabetes.

The Lean & Green Diet is also a natural method of losing weight. The main idea behind the diet is to eat more vegetables while still gaining nutrients and proteins from the foods that a person eats. Green vegetables are packed with vitamins, minerals, proteins, and other nutrients to help a person stay healthy and fit. There are many benefits to taking up the Lean & Green Diet which include better digestion, more energy from food, weight loss, lower risk of obesity/diabetes, and more.

This diet does not contain any fats or oil in it which will prevent a person from having cholesterol or heart problems in the future. A person might not be able to follow the diet 100% but they will still have a good amount of vegetables and protein. A person that is following this type of diet should avoid drinking and eating too much sugar. This will help them to maintain their weight, gain more energy and also prevent fat oxidation.

MEASUREMENT CONVERSION

COOKING CONVERSION TABLE

VOLUME MEASUREMENTS

US TO METRIC (Temperature)

°F	°C	Gas Mark
250	121	0.5
275	135	1
300	149	2
325	163	3
350	177	4
375	191	5
400	204	6
425	218	7
450	232	8
475	246	9
520	270	10

US TO METRIC (Volume)

CUP (US)	Fl. Ounces (US)	Tablespoon (TBSP-US)	Teaspoon (TSP-US)	Millilitres (ml)
1	8	16	48	237
¾	6	12	36	177
2/3	5	11	32	158
½	4	8	24	118
1/3	3	5	16	79
¼	2	4	12	59
1/8	1	2	6	30
1/16	½	1	3	15

2 CUPS (US) = 1 PINT (US)
2 CUPS (UK) = 1 PINT (UK)

METRIC TO US

°C	°F
120	248
140	284
160	320
180	356
200	392
220	428
240	464
260	500
280	536

IMPERIAL (UK) TO METRIC

CUP (UK)	Fl. Ounces (UK)	Tablespoon (TBSP-UK)	Teaspoon (TSP-UK)	Millilitres (ml)
1	10	16	48	284
¾	7.5	12	36	213
2/3	6.7	11	32	189
½	5	8	24	142
1/3	3.3	5	16	95
¼	2.5	4	12	71
1/8	1.25	2	6	36
1/16	0.625	1	3	18

Litre	Gallon (US)	Gallon (UK)	Cup (US)	Cup (UK)
3.785	1	0.833	15.77	13.32
4.546	1.2	1	18.94	16
1	0.26	0.22	4.167	3.52
0.24	0.063	0.053	1	0.844
0.28	0.075	0.062	1.183	1

WEIGHT MEASUREMENTS

Kilogram	Pounds	Ounces
1	2.204	35.27
0.454	1	16

Copyright © Gav's Kitchen

INDEX

Air Fried Beef Jerky	124
Air Fried Pot Roast	125
Air Fried Riblets	124
Air Fried Tasty Eggplant	129
Air Fryer Bell Peppers	129
Air Fryer Catfish with Cajun Seasoning	127
Air Fryer Garlic-Lime Shrimp Kebabs	128
Air Fryer Italian Pork Chops	124
Air Fryer Sushi Roll	127
Alkaline Blueberry Muffins	39
Alkaline Blueberry Spelt Pancakes	39
Almond Butter Fudge	90
Amazing Low Carb Shrimp Lettuce Wraps.	56
Ancho Tilapia on Cauliflower Rice	47
Ancho Tilapia On Cauliflower Rice	47
Apple Crisp	92
Apple Pancakes	107
Apple Salad Sandwich	105
Artichoke Soup	113
Arugula, Strawberry, & Orange Salad	108
Asian Cabbage Salad	121
Asian Green Beans	130
Asparagus & Crabmeat Frittata	46
Avocado Dip	101
Avocado Pudding	86
Avocado Taco Boat	96
Bacon & Chicken Patties	78
Bacon Cheeseburger	47
Bacon Wrapped Asparagus	49
Bacon-Wrapped Asparagus	49
Baked Beef Zucchini	68
Baked Chicken Fajitas	64
Baked Tuna with Asparagus	68
Balsamic Cabbage	17
Bananas in Nut Cups	104
Berry Mojito	19
Best Chia Pudding	84
Biscuit Pizza	37
Blue Cheese Chicken Wedges	60
Blueberry Muffins	35; 39; 89
Bok Choy and Butter Sauce	18
Bounty Bars	87
Broccoli Blue Cheese Soup	115
Broccoli Cheese Waffles	82
Broccoli Egg Bake	44
Broccoli Salad	72; 117
Brownie Bites	32
Brownie Peanut Butter Pudding	25
Brownie Pudding	25
Buckwheat Granola	106
Buttermilk Ice Cream Shake	105
Buttermilk Shake	105
Cabbage and Radishes Mix	16
California Soup	110
Cantaloupe Orange Milk Shakes	106
Caramel Crunch Parfait	24
Caramel Macchiato Frappe	22
Cashew Yogurt Bowl	41
Cauliflower Breakfast Casserole	42
Cauliflower, Spinach, and Cheese Soup	111
Celery and Green Beans Mix	101
Chard Omelet	45
Cheddar Bacon Burst	78
Cheese and Onion on Bagel	104
Cheese Broccoli Fritters	129
Cheese on Rye Bread	106
Cheesy Cauliflower Soup	110
Cheesy Onion Soup	114
Cheesy Scrambled Tofu	41
Cherry Dessert	93
Cherry Mocha Popsicles	23
Chia Pudding	86
Chia Seed Pudding	26
Chicken & Turkey Meatloaf	79
Chicken and Mushrooms	97
Chicken Broccoli Salad with Avocado Dressing	72
Chicken Cacciatore	71
Chicken Cheese Quiche	44
Chicken Enchilada Bake	98
Chicken Goulash	79
Chili Mango and Watermelon Salsa	97
Chocolate Almond Butter Brownie	89
Chocolate Berry Parfait	25
Chocolate Cake Fries	26
Chocolate Cherry Cookie	91
Chocolate Coconut Pie	24
Chocolate Crunch Cookies	28
Chocolate Frappe	22
Chocolate Frosty	87
Chocolate Haystacks	32
Chocolate Popsicle	88
Chocolate Shake	20
Chocolate Whoopie Pies	31
Cinnamon Coconut Porridge	48
Classic Low Carb Cobb Salad	57
Coconut Pancakes	40
Coconut Smoothie	19
Coriander Artichokes	16
Corner-Filling Soup	111
Cottage Cheese Hotcake	45
Crab Cakes	51
Cream of Mushroom Soup	116
Cream of Potato Soup	114
Creamy Low Carb Cream of Mushroom Soup	53
Creamy Low Carb Cream Of Mushroom Soup	53
Creamy Low Carb Zucchini Alfredo	55
Creamy Penne	74
Crisp Summer Cucumber Salad	123
Crunch Sandwich Cookies	30
Crunchy Cauliflower Salad	122

Crunchy Quinoa Meal	40
Cucumber Container with Spices and Greek Yogurt	75
Cucumber Sandwich Bites	99
Cucumber Tomato Chopped Salad	120
Curried Pumpkin Soup	113
Curried Tuna Salad	131
Delicious Brownie Bites	88
Delicious Instant Pot Keto Buffalo Chicken Soup	53
Delicious Low Carb Chicken Caesar Salad	55
Devil Eggs	46
Difficulty: Easy	51
Easy Cheese Egg Bake	43
Easy Keto Chicken Soup	53
Egg & Bacon Cups	44
Egg Avocado Salad	121
Egg drop Soup	110
Eggnog	22
Eggplant Dip	100
Fennel Wild Rice Risotto	71
Feta and Pesto Wrap	104
Feta Artichoke Dip	100
Fiery Jalapeno Poppers	77
Fish Finger Sandwich	128
Flavorful Keto Taco Soup	52
French Toast Sticks	26
Fresh Green Grape Salad	82
Fudge Balls	27
Garlic Chicken Balls	76
Garlic Kale	101
Garlicky Tomato Chicken Casserole	70
Ginger Kale	102
Gingerbread Biscotti	85
Gingersnap Cookies	29
Gluten-Free Pancakes	33
Grandma's Rice	67
Greek Roasted Fish	70
Greek Style Quesadillas	73
Greek Tuna Salad Bites	99
Green Bean Casserole	15
Green Beans	17; 101
Green Beans Rice	101
Grilled Ham & Cheese	58
Grilled Salmon with Pineapple Salsa	65
Grilled Salmon With Pineapple Salsa	65
Healthy Air Fryer Tuna Patties	128
Hearty Fruit Salad	83
Hemp Seed Porridge	35
Herbed Radish Sauté	17
Herbed Roasted Chicken Breasts	73
High Protein Salad	119
Hot Chocolate	21; 23
I Love Bacon'	61
Jalapeno Breakfast Casserole	43
Jalapeno Lentil Burgers	66
Jarlsberg Lunch Omelet	77
Kale & Mushroom Frittata	108
Kale and Walnuts	18
Kale Chips	16
Kale, Apple, & Cranberry Salad	108
Keto Cheesy Broccoli Soup	55
Keto Zucchini Pizza	50
Lamb Stuffed Avocado	69
Lasagna Spaghetti Squash	60
Lean and Green Chicken Pesto Pasta	38
Lean and Green Crockpot Chili	109
Lean and Green Smoothie 1	37
Lean and Green Smoothie 2	38
Lemon Dill Trout	61
Lemon Greek Salad	117
Lemongrass Prawns	49
Light Paprika Moussaka	74
Low Carb Black Beans Chili Chicken	51
Low Carb Parmesan Chicken Meatballs	126
Marinated Chicken Breasts	73
Marinated Eggs	97
Marinated Veggie Salad	118
Mashed Garlic Turnips	59
Matcha Pancakes	107
Meatballs Curry	61
Medifast Rolls	92
Mediterranean Burrito	75
Mediterranean Chickpea Salad	66
Mediterranean Salad	119
Mexican-Style Air Fryer Stuffed Chicken Breasts	125
Mini Mac in a Bowl	36
Mini Zucchini Bites	34
Mint chocolate pudding cookies	81
Mint Cookies	29
Mixed Vegetables with Chicken	125
Monkey Salad	77
Mozzarella Sticks	69
Mushroom & Spinach Omelet	33
Oatmeal Cookies	28
Oh so good' Salad	60
Olive Soup	116
Open-Face Egg Sandwiches with Cilantro-Jalapeño Spread	38
Optavia Granola	90
Orange Chicken Wings	127
Pan Fried Salmon	65
Parmesan Asparagus	102
Parmesan Zucchini Rounds	15
Pea Salad	120
Peanut Butter Bites	27
Peanut Butter Brownie	91
Peanut Butter Cookies	28
Peanut Butter Cups	92
Peanut Butter Fudge	90
Peanut Soup	112
Peppermint Mocha	21
Pesto Crackers	96
Pesto Zucchini Noodles	64
Pizza Hack	33
Plant-Powered Pancakes	36
Pork Taco Bake	63
Pork Tenderloin with Fried Bell Peppers	124
Pork with Veggies	62
Potato Carrot Salad	118
Potato Tuna Salad	119
Prosciutto Spinach Salad	59
Prosciutto Wrapped Mozzarella Balls	76
Pumpkin Balls	88
Pumpkin Frappe	21
Pumpkin Muffins	98
Pumpkin Spiced Latte	23
Quick Healthy Avocado Tuna Salad	52
Quick Keto Blt Chicken Salad	51

Quick Keto BLT Chicken Salad	51	Sweet Pumpkin Waffles	85
Quick Keto Roasted Tomato Soup	54	Swiss cheese and Broccoli Soup	115
Quinoa with Vegetables	79	Taco Casserole	54
Raspberry Ice Cream	87	Taco Salad	130
Riced Cauliflower & Curry Chicken	59	Tangy Kale Salad	122
Roasted Tomatoes	18	Tasty Low Carb Cucumber Salad	56
Salmon Burger	103	Tasty Low Carb Cucumber Salad.	56
Salmon Sandwich with Avocado and Egg	103	Tasty Onion and Cauliflower Dip	95
Sandwich Cookies	30	Tasty Pecan Pie Muffins	81
Sausage and Cheese Dip	95	Tavern Soup	115
Sausage Egg Omelet	43	Tiramisu Shake	20
Sautéd Crispy Zucchini	64	Tomato Fish Bake	70
Sautéed Crispy Zucchini	64	Turkey Caprese Meatloaf Cups	48
Scrambled Pesto Eggs	46	Turmeric Mushroom	19
Seafood Paella	72	Vanilla Avocado Popsicles	89
Shake Cake Fueling	37	Vanilla Frappe	21
Shamrock Shake	20	Vanilla Pudding	93
Smoked Salmon & Kale Scramble	107	Vanilla Shake	19; 20; 21; 22; 31
Smooth Peanut Butter Cream	86	Vegan Waffles with Kale	83
Snap Pea Salad	120	Veggie Fritters	99
Snickerdoodles	31	Walnut Crunch Banana Bread	35
Soap De Frijoles Negros	112	Warm Chorizo Chickpea Salad	66
Spicy Asian Brussels Sprouts	130	Wasabi Tuna Asian Salad	117
Spicy Red Cabbage	102	White Bean Dip	100
Spinach and Artichokes Sauté	17	Whole-Wheat Blueberry Muffins	35
Spinach and Cottage Cheese Sandwich	103	Wild Rice Prawn Salad	71
Spinach Chicken	49	Yogurt Cereal Bark	27
Spinach Pie	63	Yogurt Cookie Dough	24
Sriracha-honey Chicken Wings	126	Yogurt Garlic Chicken	58
Stracciatella	111	Yogurt Trail Mix Bars	130
Stuffed Avocado	69; 95	Yummy Keto Mushroom Asparagus Frittata	57
Stuffed Bell Peppers with Quinoa	75	Yummy Lime Pie	82
Stuffed Mushrooms	50	Zucchini Bacon Bake	42
Stuffed pears with almonds	91	Zucchini Breakfast Bars	41
Sweet Cashew Cheese Spread	34	Zucchini Pasta Salad	121
Sweet Potato Bacon Mash	76	Zucchini Salmon Salad	65
Sweet Potato Muffins	84	Zucchini Spaghetti	15

Printed in Great Britain
by Amazon